Luminos is the Open Access monograph publishing program
from UC Press. Luminos provides a framework for preserving and
reinvigorating monograph publishing for the future and increases
the reach and visibility of important scholarly work. Titles published
in the UC Press Luminos model are published with the same high
standards for selection, peer review, production, and marketing as
those in our traditional program. www.luminosoa.org

Fencing in AIDS

Fencing in AIDS

Gender, Vulnerability, and Care in Papua New Guinea

———

Holly Wardlow

UNIVERSITY OF CALIFORNIA PRESS

University of California Press
Oakland, California

Suggested citation: Wardlow, H. *Fencing in AIDS: Gender, Vulnerability, and Care in Papua New Guinea*. Oakland: University of California Press, 2020. DOI: https://doi.org/10.1525/luminos.94

Names: Wardlow, Holly, author.
Title: Fencing in AIDS : gender, vulnerability, and care in Papua
   New Guinea / Holly Wardlow.
Description: Oakland, California : University of California Press, [2020] |
   Includes bibliographical references and index.
Identifiers: LCCN 2020010287 (print) | LCCN 2020010288 (ebook) |
   ISBN 9780520355514 (paperback) | ISBN 9780520975941 (ebook)
Subjects: LCSH: AIDS (Disease) in women—Papua New Guinea—
   Tari Distric—Case studies.
Classification: LCC RA643.86.P262 W37 2020 (print) |
   LCC RA643.86.P262 (ebook) | DDC 362.19697/92009953—dc23
LC record available at https://lccn.loc.gov/2020010287
LC ebook record available at https://lccn.loc.gov/2020010288

29   28   27   26   25   24   23   22   21   20
10   9   8   7   6   5   4   3   2   1

CONTENTS

LIST OF ILLUSTRATIONS

MAP

FIGURES

ACKNOWLEDGMENTS

This book is based on research carried out over almost ten years, and there are consequently many, many individuals and organizations to thank for their assistance, friendship, and support. As always, my deepest thanks go to Mary Tamia and June Pogaya, my beloved besties in Tari, who have shared everything with me—stories, food, families, insights, laughter, tears, fear, and, fury. I am also deeply thankful for Jacinta Hayabe's friendship since 1996. During our many long, cigarette-filled, late-night conversations, she proved an invaluable interlocutor and especially helped me understand the complex political field of women's groups in the region. I am grateful to Michael Parali, Luke Magala, Ken Angobe, and Thomas Mindibi, the four wonderful men who worked as my field assistants in 2004, were brave enough to pose forthright questions about love, sex, marriage, extramarital relationships, and HIV to their peers, and had no compunction about telling me when interview questions were problematic.

My deepest condolences go to the family of Joseph Warai, who directed the Community Based Health Care (CBHC) NGO in the mid 2000s and was very supportive of my 2004 research project. Joseph and the whole CBHC team persevered in delivering health promotion and income-generating projects to people in the Tari area during a desperate and precarious period, and they were a source of hope and inspiration for many. I was also sad to learn that Sister Pauline Agilo had died. She was a comfort to many people living with HIV and AIDS, and especially helped people as best she could in the pre-antiretroviral era.

During my research stints in 2010, 2011, 2012, and 2013, a number of health workers assisted me by telling patients about my research and asking them if they were interested in being interviewed. They also, with the permission of patients, allowed me to observe some of their counselling sessions, and they shared with me their concerns about patients' living situations and about the sometimes unreliable availability of antiretrovirals and other essential medicines in Tari. I am especially grateful for Margaret Parale's friendship and assistance during this research. Employees of the Oil Search Health Foundation also assisted in recruiting participants for me, and provided me with useful data about Tari's HIV prevalence. Jethiro Harrison and Ruben Enoch were University of Papua New Guinea student interns with me in Tari for a few weeks in 2013. Among other things, they helped me to understand the powerful allure of Port Moresby that can attach itself to those who have lived there and attract other people when they return to rural areas. I am also grateful to the staff of Médecins sans frontières in Tari who were so generous to me, especially when my guesthouse did not have water or electricity.

I feel profoundly lucky to belong to the Department of Anthropology at the University of Toronto, where I have wonderful and brilliant colleagues, whose ideas have influenced mine. I am also grateful to have been part of the "Love, Marriage, and HIV" multi-sited research team. Jennifer Hirsch, Dan Smith, Harriet Phinney, Shanti Parikh, and Constance Nathanson are remarkable researchers and wonderful friends, and it was a blessing and joy to be able to work collaboratively on a research project with them.

I am very thankful to the organizations that funded the research projects that went into this book, the U.S. National Institutes of Health (grant #1 RO1 HD41724) and the Canadian Social Science and Humanities Research Council (Standard Research Grant #331985). I am grateful, too, for the affiliations granted to me during my research to the Papua New Guinea Institute of Medical Research (2004) and the Papua New Guinea National Research Institute (2011–13). I also thank the University of Toronto, and especially our Faculty Association (UTFA): because of my accumulated annual PERA (professional expense reimbursement allowance) I was able to provide the subvention subsidy to make this book open access.

Finally, my family has given me unstinting love and encouragement. I am especially thankful for my partner, Ken MacDonald, who was with me in Tari in 2013 and provided a number of photographs for this book, and my mother, Diane Wardlow, who read the book manuscript at least twice and has always been an enthusiastic supporter. I also thank my niece, Natalia Sierra-Wardlow, who is the delight of my life and who asks thought-provoking questions about Papua New Guinea and book writing.

Introduction

"We Are No Longer Fenced In"

I sometimes find myself thinking about Julai,[1] and I wonder where she is now. I met her in 2004 when I was doing research in Tari on married women's risk of contracting HIV. Initially an interviewee, then a recruiter of other women for me to interview, Julai eventually became a friend. She is sweet, funny, and frank, and I was drawn to her openhearted, open-minded ways. I often worried about her, because she is generous to a fault. One of her preferred ways of earning money was to buy cartons of cigarettes wholesale and then sell the cigarettes singly for a profit, a very common strategy in Tari. But she was forever giving cigarettes away to her *besties* (close friends), or smoking them herself, and was never able to get ahead.

When I met Julai, she was separated from her husband, who had left a few years before to find work at a gold mine in another province. He had stopped sending money or messages home, but she heard rumors that he was sleeping around, and then learned that he was living with another woman. Enraged at being abandoned and left to care for their son on her own, she had begun having sex with other men. At first motivated by anger and a desire to even the score—"If he can fool around, so can I [*Em inap faul raun, bai mi tu faul raun*]," she said—her philandering came to be driven by other sentiments: feeling flattered by a powerful or wealthy man's interest in her, needing money to pay for her son's schooling, or thinking a man might make a good replacement husband. She talked about three regular partners during the six months I was in Tari in 2004, as well as a number of one-off inter-actions with other men. I did my best to educate her about HIV, and I gave her condoms, both for her own use and to sell. (Condoms were not readily available at Tari Hospital or in local stores at that time, so I made periodic visits to the National AIDS Council offices in Port Moresby, Papua New Guinea's capital city, and returned with large cartons of them, which I gave to field assistants, friends, and people I interviewed.) Julai told me she was an experienced and regular, if not scrupulous, condom user, but I still worried.

In 2013, Julai informed me that she was HIV-positive. Her husband had moved back home a few years before, and although he had been away for most of the previous seven years, he was furious about what he'd heard of her sexual activity in his absence. Julai showed me pornographic images he had sent her by cell phone, images that were intended to insult, not titillate. They showed one stick figure fucking another from behind (mobile phones were relatively new at that time in Tari, and most people's phones in Tari were quite basic, with limited data) and made me laugh, but Julai was deeply offended. She was saving the messages for a possible future village court case. Shaming people in public by talking in sexually disparaging or humiliating ways about their bodies—referred to as *diskraibim* (describe) in Tok Pisin (Wardlow 2006a: 99)—was still a compensable offense in Tari, and although there were contentious debates about whether mobile phone messages counted, Julai was accumulating evidence just in case.

Julai and her husband had had sex during the rare times he visited Tari. They were still officially married (no bridewealth had been returned), and Julai sometimes seemed to hope that they could repair their relationship. She decided to get tested for HIV when she learned that he had tested positive, but she did not know whether he was the one who had infected her or one of her other partners. Despite testing positive at Tari Hospital, she was not put on antiretroviral medication (hereafter referred to as ARVs or ART): her CD4 count—a measure of immune system strength—was too high and she seemed healthy and strong.[2] She said that she had been told to return in a year to have her CD4 count tested again.

I knew that if she had gone to the small AIDS Care Centre, just a twenty-minute walk from Tari Hospital, she would have been put on ARVs immediately. The Centre didn't have a CD4 machine and had adopted the policy of "test and start"— that is, putting everyone who tested positive on treatment. However, Julai firmly rejected my suggestion that she go there. In fact, she was relieved about her results and felt she'd been given a reprieve—if the hospital staff said she didn't have to be on medication and didn't have to return for a whole year, surely that must be good news. She was not going to let herself worry unnecessarily about being sick. A few months later, after I had returned to Canada, clan warfare broke out where she lived, Julai and her son had to flee, and they were now cut off from the hospital. I have been unable to get information about her since.

· · ·

When HIV arrives in a place, it encounters a specific political, economic, social, and discursive terrain. It enters at a particular historical moment, and the nature of this moment—whether politically placid or tumultuous, economically thriving or bleak—can shape both how the virus moves through a community and how its spread is understood and acted upon. In the case of Tari, HIV arrived during a time of immense turmoil and change, from a period of state abandonment, economic decline, and post-election violence in the late 1990s and early 2000s, to the founding of a new province and the development of an immense new liquefied natural gas project in the early 2010s. When HIV arrives in a place, it might also be said to encounter a particular moral terrain, in the sense that infection may be attributed to moral transgressions, and people living with HIV may feel compelled to conduct themselves in particular ways in order to protect themselves from moral judgment or demonstrate their ethical intentions to others.

Among the Huli, the customary cultural group of the Tari area, the fence is an important element of both the physical and moral terrain and is often invoked to explain the spread of HIV: "We are no longer fenced in," many people lamented, when I asked why AIDS was prevalent in the region. Real, material fences are said to facilitate proper moral behavior by minimizing temptation (Wardlow 2006a: 40), and deep ditches and stands of tall trees and bushes often surround family properties. These are said to shield the residents and their belongings from the covetous gaze of others, while also protecting the latter from acquisitiveness and the temptation to steal. Customary rules and prohibitions are conceptualized as figurative fences: by confining people and limiting their behavior, they create a moral space in which they can flourish. Just as fields or pigs need to be fenced in so that they can fulfill their proper purpose of growing and thriving, so people too need to be "fenced in" so that they can properly fulfill their sociomoral purpose of developing, laboring, marrying, and reproducing. The fence in this idiom is at once disciplinary, protective, nurturing, and generative of proper purpose.

In asserting, "We are no longer fenced in," Huli mean that their lives are now less morally ordered, because the customs of the past no longer constrain and compel behavior. Like pigs that have escaped their enclosures, Huli say of themselves, they are now free of their traditional customs, but they lack purpose, meaning, or direction. In particular, they are no longer guided and constrained by precolonial moral knowledge regarding gendered conduct and sexual practice. Because HIV is often perceived through this self-chastising nostalgic lens, Huli discourse about HIV is always also discourse about gender propriety, Huli customs, the consequences of, but also failures to achieve, "development," and the place of the Huli within the nation-state. Fencing in AIDS (that is, preventing its spread), people say, requires more than medicine: it requires fencing in people, which for some means convincing people to be better Christians, and for others means recognizing the benefits of Huli customs and trying to revitalize them. Both of these are seen as increasingly difficult, however, in a context of high mobility, resource extraction, and the failure of the government to provide needed services or to prevent tribal fighting and crime.

In this book I focus specifically on women's encounters with HIV—as pathogen, site of family and governmental discipline, and affective and moral experience. The phrase "the feminization of AIDS" has commonly been used to refer to women's disproportionate infection with HIV, and it is shorthand for the fact that female sex (specifically, female reproductive physiology) and female gender (a relation of power) interact to make girls and women more vulnerable than men. "The biological make-up of the female body only goes some way to explain the feminisation of the epidemic: the central meaning of the term derives from social and cultural explanations as to why women are more vulnerable to HIV infection," Sophie Harman explains (2011: 2014–15). Globally, these social and cultural explanations include: lower educational levels; less access to paid employment; economic and sometimes reputational dependency on men; less control over money, land, and other assets; less ability to control whether, when, and how sex takes place; and greater vulnerability to sexual and family violence, as well as the inability to safely exit from violent relationships.

I conceptualize the feminization of the epidemic in more expansive terms, examining not only women's vulnerability to infection but also the ways that they are interpellated by AIDS awareness programs as both victims and "unsanitary subjects" (Briggs with Mantini 2003), and how they are perceived by family and community members as harboring unknowable, and perhaps dangerous, intentions after testing HIV-positive. Each chapter shows how being gendered female shapes every aspect of HIV, from being trafficked to landowners at a nearby gold mine, to being admonished for incompetent sexual hygiene during AIDS education workshops, to being considered morally suspect once diagnosed HIV-positive. Elements of Julai's story—her husband's long absence at a mine and his marrying an additional wife while there, her consequent anger and economic insecurity, her quite good access to ARVs once she tested positive, and her determination not to worry about HIV, even if this meant delaying treatment—all speak to important elements of women's experiences of HIV in Tari. The six remaining sections of this Introduction provide important background about HIV/AIDS in Tari: the region's tumultuous recent history, Huli gender ideologies and practices, the complexities and ambiguities of HIV prevalence data in Papua New Guinea, how AIDS has been interpreted and understood in Tari, the research methods and participants, and an overview of the book's chapters.

TARI'S RECENT HISTORY

Tari occupies a special place in both Papua New Guinea's economy and its national imaginary, and this makes it an important site for doing research into HIV/AIDS. Papua New Guinea is heavily reliant on the exploitation of minerals, oil, and natural gas, and Tari is centrally located between world-class gold mines to the north and west (in Porgera and Tabubil), as well as significant oil and natural gas projects to the south (most recently, ExxonMobil's new liquefied natural gas project, commonly referred to as the PNG LNG or simply the LNG). The Huli, one of the largest cultural groups in Papua New Guinea, have a history dating back to

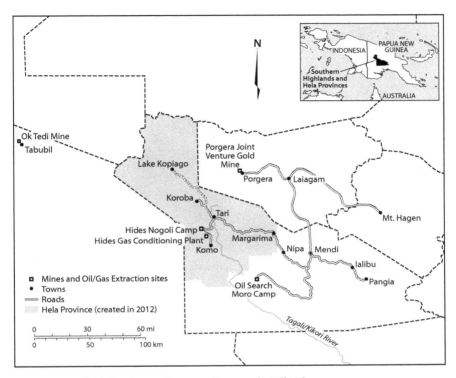

MAP 1. Map of Hela Province and surrounding areas by Bill Nelson.

the 1970s of male migration out of Tari to work on plantations and at mine sites in other provinces (Harris 1972, Ward 1990, Lehmann 2002). Because of this, Huli often claim that they have played an outsized role in the economic development of the nation. Furthermore, they sometimes claim to be the rightful inheritors of Papua New Guinea, destined to rule it. This kind of hubris does not make them beloved in the nation.

As discussed above, fences are deeply meaningful to Huli—materially, metaphorically, and morally—and I have always found that the long, tall fence enclosing the airport is a telling indicator of the state of affairs in Tari. Like most highland towns in Papua New Guinea, Tari began as an airstrip with a few colonial administrative buildings alongside it. It has grown, of course, but the long runway is still in the center, with stores, the main market, government buildings, a police station, and public servant housing on one side, and the hospital, police barracks, and more housing on the other. The runway is long enough to accommodate large commercial planes, and walking its perimeter takes almost an hour. Throughout the day, people walk around it to get from one side to the other—women carrying produce to market, patients trying to get to the hospital, and so on. When I arrived in Tari

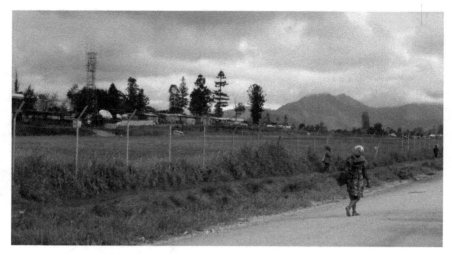

FIGURE 1. Woman walking alongside the Tari airport fence. Photo by author.

in 2004, after an absence of seven years, I found the airport fence in a shocking state of disrepair. Sections had been ripped out, goats and sheep often wandered freely around the airfield by day, and at night some people sprinted across it, going through the broken sections rather than walk all the way around. People raucously exchanged stories about the police suddenly roaring onto the airstrip in their four-wheel-drive trucks, high beams on, chasing people back and forth, acting as if they would run them down, and then finally hauling them off to jail for trespassing on government property. "But why should we respect the government's fence?" people grumbled. "Schools and health centers are closed, the police have run away, the politicians are too afraid to come here, and we only ever see the bellies of the planes flying overhead—we have no money to ever go inside one."

This last sentence sums up Tari's plight in 2004. As discussed in more detail in chapter 2, Papua New Guinea's Southern Highlands Province, of which Tari was then a part, had experienced failed elections in 2002. People had been forced to vote for particular candidates, ballot boxes were stolen at gunpoint from the Tari police station and dumped into a river, and violence was widespread, resulting in a number of deaths (Haley and May 2007). Government services had been declining before the elections, and they worsened after them, in part because the failed elections meant that there was no provincial government: public servants weren't paid, government offices in Mendi, the provincial capital, were abandoned and then ransacked, and gradually schools and health centers closed throughout the province as their staffs fled the region.

When people in Tari talk about this period (approximately 2000–2004), they speak of "living in fear"—fear of armed holdups on the roads, of home invasion, of being abducted and raped by gangs, of being badly injured and there being no healthcare—but they also talk about the people who didn't run away. They remember, for example, which hospital staff continued to work, despite not being paid and running out of essential medicines. And they remember the Catholic nuns, both national and expatriate, who remained when other missionaries and public servants fled. People warmly recall, for example, the tough-minded nun-headmistress of Tari Secondary School, who kept the school open when all other high schools in the province closed, even when a gang of young men drove onto the campus and abducted female students out of their dorms at gunpoint and threatened to kill her and the teachers who resisted.

During the six months I spent in Tari in 2004, things improved somewhat. A caretaker government had been installed until new elections could be held, and, to most people's profound relief, one of Papua New Guinea's mobile squads (special police units assigned to crisis areas and known for their aggressive policing tactics) had been assigned to Tari to restore order. Some schools reopened, there were sometimes nurses working in the outpatient ward at Tari Hospital, and a few small stores sold basic goods, such as rice, canned fish, salt, and soap. A small community-based development project had been established to help families grow and sell coffee and to provide them with chickens, ducks, and water tanks (Vail 2007). The Porgera Joint Venture gold mine (PJV) had opened a small community affairs office in Tari, providing some employment, as well as funds for youth groups and women's groups. There was still no electricity, however, and armed holdups on the roads were common. When I returned for a few weeks in 2006, things were again much better. Schools had reopened, and more staff had returned to the hospital.

This context is important, because it was during this turbulent period—the late 1990s and early 2000s—when many of the HIV-positive women I interviewed from 2011 to 2013 were infected. As I discuss in the first three chapters of this book, many were infected by husbands working at mines in the region, some were infected through selling sex, and a couple of them were infected when raped. The number of women exchanging sex for money increased noticeably during this period, and hospital records also indicate a dramatic surge in sexual violence, which I discuss in chapter 2. Moreover, because of the breakdown in health services, the difficulties in getting any medical supplies to Tari Hospital, and the reluctance of hospital staff to distribute them, there were very few condoms available.

When I returned in 2010, the Tari airport fence had been completely rebuilt, there were now signs at regular intervals warning people not to climb over it onto the runway, and a large area at one end had been closed off and was secured by guards hired to protect PNG LNG construction materials. There was no more running across the airfield at night. PNG LNG managerial staff had taken over every possible hotel and guesthouse in Tari and Mendi and were flown daily back and forth to LNG project sites by helicopter. Eighteen-wheelers carrying LNG supplies drove through Tari day and night, raising clouds of red dust. One entrepreneurial woman had built a large guesthouse specifically for workers sub-contracted to the LNG project, and although the rooms were small and spartan, they rented for U.S.$100–200 a night; tractor-trailers were lined up nose to tail outside, and the guesthouse was always full.

The construction or development phase of a gas project, particularly in a remote area with little existing infrastructure, is a hugely labor-intensive undertaking. In the case of the LNG, it was expected to have a 14,000-person workforce during its peak construction phase. Roads had to be constructed; compounds had to be built for the laborers who would build the gas-conditioning plant and drill sites; landowners had be identified, compensated, and relocated. Six hundred licensed truck drivers had to be hired to transport heavy machinery and supplies (and, at the start of the construction phase, the whole of Papua New Guinea only had four hundred, most of whom already had jobs working in other industries; the LNG project lured many of them away by offering much higher salaries). And even more local people were hired as cleaners, cooks, launderers, and security guards.

Most spectacularly, the longest runway in Papua New Guinea had to be built near the tiny government center of Komo, at the cost of approximately U.S.$700 million, to accommodate the enormous Antonov AN-124 cargo planes scheduled to bring in the largest equipment and machinery. This runway was to be used by the project for only eighteen months, and then relinquished to the Papua New Guinea government. Given that the project was expected to generate hundreds of billions of dollars, and contracts had already been signed with Tokyo Electric and Osaka Gas in Japan, as well as with Sinopec in China, a $700 million runway that might never again be used was a reasonable expense. This runway took much longer to be built than expected because of unanticipated swampy conditions. As it was cagily explained to me by a high-level manager involved in the project, "the airstrip keeps sinking into the ground." And while the delay created a great deal of anxiety at the national and international levels about whether ExxonMobil would meet its deadline for exporting the gas (it did), it was a source of delight at the local level, because it generated ever more employment and income: new rock quarries had to be identified and acquired, and new truck drivers had to be hired to transport more and more rock in order to build up the sinking runway. It was a tremendously busy and exciting time for Tari, with plentiful employment after a long period of almost none.[3]

As exciting, and largely because of the LNG project, the new Hela Province was being created from a portion of what had been Southern Highlands Province. Huli have longed for their own province ever since Papua New Guinea gained independence in 1975; many speak of it as cosmologically ordained (Haley 2007), and others claim it was promised to them by Michael Somare, first prime minister of the country. Some people literally danced in the streets with joy as they prepared for the new province's inaugural celebrations in 2010. A politician who was key to the negotiations told me that he had informed ExxonMobil executives that

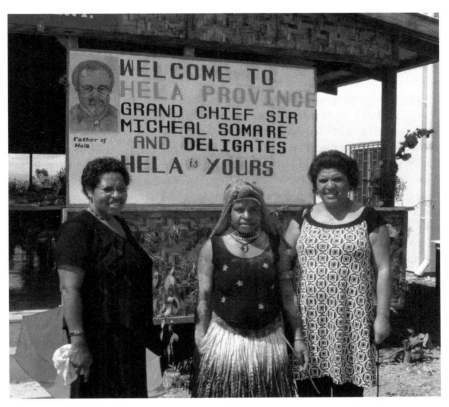

FIGURE 2. Women leaders Veronica Lunnie Payawi, Mary Tamia, and Marilyn Tabagua celebrate the creation of Hela Province. Photo by author.

he would block the LNG project's approval if they did not support the creation of Hela Province in whatever ways they could; thus, the fates of the LNG project and Hela Province were intertwined, and ultimately they were co-creations. The demand for Hela was motivated by a desire to transform Huli territory from a zone peripheral to and remote from state power into its own center of power, with control over resources, opportunities, and services. And what its creation meant most immediately was even more jobs: Tari needed to be readied for its new role as a provincial capital, and international NGOs like Médecins sans frontières (MSF) and Population Services International (PSI), never present in Tari before, arrived to establish humanitarian and development projects.

It was in this context that antiretroviral treatment (ARVs) became widely available in the Tari area. Although ARVs had been available since 2007 at Tari Hospital and the nearby Catholic AIDS Care Centre, the LNG project helped improve access immensely. Oil Search Ltd., the primary joint venture partner with Exxon-Mobil in the LNG project, made HIV education, testing, and treatment in Hela a prominent part of its corporate social responsibility portfolio, and it invested in training staff, improving data collection and monitoring, and upgrading the network of small health-care centers throughout Hela. In the space of two or three years, HIV-related services went from being available only if you could get to Tari town to being widely accessible.

The LNG project also affected how Huli were viewed by others in the nation-state. The Huli have long had a reputation for being aggressive, and, since the mid 1990s, when I first started doing fieldwork in the Tari area, I have sometimes heard them described by other Papua New Guineans as "primitive," "violent," and "unciv-ilized." At the same time, I have often also heard the Huli lauded by other Papua New Guineans, usually men, because "they have maintained their traditions when the rest of us have abandoned them." What these admirers usually mean by "tradi-tions" is the Huli practice of gender separation: as they do to a much smaller extent now, in the past, husbands and wives lived in separate houses, sometimes quite far from each other, and men farmed their own sweet potato fields and cooked for themselves. Since the LNG project, however, Huli are more often imagined as wealthy, arrogant, wasteful, and as having abandoned the customs that once made them worthy of admiration. During the construction stage of the drilling sites and gas-conditioning plant, roughly from 2009 to 2013, Huli landowners received large sums of money through jobs, relocation packages, business start-up grants, and various other cash infusions intended to ensure that the project was not derailed by local discontent. Newly wealthy powerful Huli men flew back and forth to Port Moresby to drink, gamble, and maintain their connections with politicians tied to the project. Although these men made up a tiny segment of the Huli population, they were a very visible segment and had a significant impact on how Huli were imagined by others.

GENDER AND HIV IN TARI

I originally envisaged this project as a comparison of men's and women's expe-riences of HIV vulnerability and treatment. However, because so few men were seeking testing and treatment between 2010 and 2013, I did not have enough inter-views, conversations, or participant-observation data with men to feel comfortable making many generalizations about them. Moreover, I cut short four of the eight formal interviews I had with men because I felt they were too sick to continue (this was not true of any of my interviews with women). Most of these men had refused to seek help until they were so unwell that others made the choice for them, and two of them died over the course of my research, although none of the women did. The reluctance of men to seek HIV testing, and their typically much later entry into care, is a widespread global problem (Shand et al. 2014), and is attributed to a range of factors, including men's discomfort with hospital spaces, which often feel to them like female spaces, populated mostly by female nurses and patients, as well as men's aversion to acknowledging vulnerability or dependency. It may also be that becoming an "AIDS patient"—with its expectations of pharmaceutical obedience, absolute sobriety, and sexual abstemiousness—is experienced by them as relinquishing masculine identity, and thus something to be avoided (cf. Mfecane 2011).

Despite my comparatively thin data about men, some clear themes did emerge. For one thing, Huli men were more fearful than women of being ostracized because of HIV and less likely to disclose their status. They feared very material consequences, such as clan members using a man's HIV-positive status as a pretext for trying to appropriate his land. And men were more likely to express deep unhappiness about there being no cure, and thus were more likely to experiment with alternative treatments and to make their own decisions about whether to follow the antiretroviral regimen as instructed. There are, in short, some interesting gendered comparisons to be made. In the end, however, I decided to focus primarily on women, though of course it is impossible to discuss HIV vulnerability and treatment without discussing women's relationships with men (as wives, mothers, daughters, sisters, sexual partners, etc.).

As mentioned above, I've heard Papua New Guineans from other regions, especially men, speak of the Huli with admiration for what they see as their tenacious adherence to tradition, especially the separation of men and women into different sociospatial domains, often underpinned and legitimized by ideologies about the dangers that women pose to men (Glasse 1968, 1974; Frankel 1980, 1986; Goldman 1983; Clark 1993; Wardlow 2006a). When I first began researching Huli women's lives in the mid 1990s, in a rural area north of Tari, many married couples lived in separate houses, sometimes only 25–50 yards apart, but sometimes on clan territories quite distant from each other. A few young unmarried men I knew made a point of growing their own food and eschewing contact with women, even walking alongside of footpaths so as not to tread on female footprints. Nevertheless, even in the 1990s, it was clear that things were changing dramatically. In point of fact, only one-third of married men did not live with their wives, according to a survey done by one of my field assistants, and most men whose houses were old planned to build new, larger houses with the intention of living in them with their wives and children. As reasons for this change, they sometimes said they wanted to be good Christians (Wardlow 2014) or wanted the convenience of living with a wife (e.g., they no longer wanted to cook for themselves). In sum, despite prevailing discourses about the dangers of excessive contact between the genders, most Huli married couples today live and eat together, and people are far more comfortable with heterosociality.

That said, Huli people also regularly debate whether changes like spousal cohabitation are having beneficial or detrimental effects on Huli society. Does spousal cohabitation cause men to become physically and morally weaker? Does it cause more fighting between spouses than in the past? Clearly shaken by it, one of my male field assistants described the following incident during one of our team meetings in 2004:

> Recently, as part of a bridewealth celebration, I was invited to eat pork in a clan men's house, and I got inside and realized that the men were eating the pig's stomach and intestines (organs traditionally eaten only by women and children). I'd never seen men eating pig intestines before, and I was shocked and disgusted. And I worried that men in my generation are becoming like women.

He added:

> Doing these interviews with men (about their marriages and extramarital experiences) gives me the same feeling—that men are becoming like women. [In what way?] Too many of them talk about being unable to control their desires—desire for sex clouds their judgment and makes them confused. They are impulsive and do things that they later regret. I was always taught that only women and children are like that. Men are supposed to be single-minded; they are decisive, they are self-disciplined.

This kind of concern was expressed often—that spousal cohabitation, and increased heterosociality more generally, have corrupted proper, resolute, self-disciplined masculinity, and that the social order has eroded as a consequence.

Women's increased autonomy (freedom to go to school, to join women's groups, to walk to town and sell things at market) was also subject to critical scrutiny. Men were often unhappy that women used their freedom of movement to spend time with their female kin and friends, whom men often viewed as morally corrupting influences. This is summed up in the Huli aphorism, "The tame pigs follow the wild pigs," which refers to the observation that if domesticated pigs are not guarded carefully and manage to escape the household fence, they will run away, join herds of wild pigs, and lose any domesticated habits they had. Similarly, proper women and girls are said to be easily led by irresponsible sisters and friends into gossip, gambling, smoking, flirting, and worse. Notable here is that men, in their roles as fathers, brothers, and husbands, often see themselves as responsible for ensuring that women behave morally, and physical altercations and punitive violence often result from men's and women's disagreements about female autonomy.

In 2008, Médecins sans frontières established a project at Tari Hospital dedicated to providing surgical, medical, and psychological care for the survivors of family and sexual violence, almost all of whom, not surprisingly, were women and girls (MSF 2011). Though MSF was scrupulous in its reports and clinical interactions to frame this as a project about "family violence"—in part, I believe, so as not to antagonize local men—in practice it largely concerned men's violence against women. That an international humanitarian organization saw family/gender violence in Tari as so problematic that it decided to establish a project about it there came as a surprise to many people, spurring some confusion and much reflection.[4]

Most of the women I have interviewed since the mid 1990s have been hit by their husbands (though the frequency and severity vary enormously), and hospital records show that women suffer far more severe injuries than men do from family violence. Nevertheless, it is also the case that women are encouraged by mothers and sisters to hit their husbands if they behave in insulting or disrespectful ways, and little girls, like little boys, are encouraged to hit people who take their belongings or who hurt loved ones (Wardlow 2006a). Most of the women I have interviewed are quite proud of their readiness to engage in physical fighting when necessary, including with husbands, and they take great pleasure in giving blow-by-blow accounts of the fights they have been in. "Everyone has two hands and can fight" is a common saying. Thus, people seemed quite divided as to whether the level of violence between spouses was unusual or problematic, as the MSF project seemed to imply. In contrast, many expressed a great deal of concern about what they perceived as an increase in violence between male kin, especially brothers, due to conflicts over land and resource-extraction benefits. In other words, MSF's framing of the situation in Tari as a problem of "family and sexual violence" did not entirely overlap with how people in Tari understood the increases in interpersonal violence spurred by recent political and economic changes.

The issue of gender violence in Tari bears directly on HIV vulnerability. Much of the literature about AIDS in Papua New Guinea has emphasized gender-based violence, especially sexual violence, as being a significant factor in Papua New Guinea's epidemic (Seeley and Butcher 2006, Lepani 2008, Lewis et al. 2008, Hammar 2010, Eves 2010, Redman-MacLaren et al. 2013, Shih et al. 2017). How to theorize this violence has been a troubling question. A number of scholars have pointed to "embattled masculinities" (Jolly 2000) or "troubled masculinities," which Laura Zimmer-Tamakoshi defines as

> men's abject lack of control over the resources they need to achieve both local and global ideals of masculine social and individual power. . . . Unable to achieve community (much less global) expectations, many of today's young men feel unfairly placed in social-psychic pressure cookers of impossible expectations, feelings that may contribute to acts of compensatory violence as well as violent efforts to force others . . . to help them achieve social manhood. (Zimmer-Tamakoshi 2012: 82–83; see also Jolly 2012)

I would add that while Huli men do express anxiety and frustration about their inability to achieve the economic security they need to care for their families and to maintain the respect of their peers, such feelings are also triggered by police violence, corrupt politicians, racist mining personnel, poor social services, and lack of control over extractable resources found on their own customary land. In other words, men's frustrations may have many sources and are not always about the obstacles to achieving hegemonic masculinity. In any case, this analytic framework suggests that gender violence is a phenomenon in which women bear the brunt of men's postcolonial existential distress.

Martha Macintyre points out, however, that "aggressive masculine behavior is implicitly valued as both an expression of engagement with modernity and as an ideal of charismatic self-assertion that is transgressive, audacious and risky" (Macintyre 2008: 180). In other words, demonstrating one's readiness and capacity for violence may actually be an element of hegemonic masculinity, not a reaction to one's failure to achieve it. Macintyre urges scholars to recognize the historical "continuities in masculine embodiment and self-presentation, as both beautiful and dangerous" (181), while also cautioning that such analyses "must be then situated within the contemporary world of increasing economic inequality and mobility, as well as failures of government" (181). Margaret Jolly, for her part, has recently cautioned against making generalizations about Pacific masculinities and violence and instead emphasizes the significant generational and status differences between men, as well as the analytical importance being attuned to how masculinities are "formed and transformed" (Jolly 2016: 305) throughout history and especially in contexts of colonialism and postcolonialism (see also Biersack 2016).

I would also note that national surveys demonstrating high rates of gendered violence in Papua New Guinea date back thirty-five years (see Toft 1985). This means that at least one generation of children has grown up witnessing parental and other forms of interpersonal and gendered violence, suggesting that anthropologists and other scholars of Papua New Guinea might consider engaging with theories about intergenerational cycles of violence. Carrying out research in Tari since the 1990s has allowed me to witness the transformation of young boys traumatized by their parents' fighting—they learned when very young to hide all household axes and knives whenever the fighting started, and they often ran sobbing to neighbors' houses—into young men, some of whom now hit their wives. To my knowledge, most research about gender violence in Papua New Guinea has not inquired deeply enough into women's and men's childhoods, their parents' marriages, or how they understood the violence they witnessed and experienced when young. Finally, it is important to take into account that gendered violence occurs frequently in areas where economic insecurity, social disorder, and other kinds of violence—state and local political violence, for example—are also highly prevalent. Gendered violence is often one element or symptom of a broader environment of precarity and violence.

HIV PREVALENCE DATA IN PAPUA NEW GUINEA

The first questions people tend to ask when I tell them I do research on AIDS in Papua New Guinea are "How bad is it?" or "What percentage of people have it?" I always find myself hesitating about how to answer, because, until very recently, data for Papua New Guinea were scarce and poor. Prevalence—the proportion of a population that has an illness condition—is the primary way we know a disease at the population level; it tells us the extent of the problem. And, when we search the internet to obtain information about a disease, we expect to be able to find a table that at least appears to establish prevalence definitively. However, the numbers in those tables are not easily achieved—they require health service infrastructure, widespread testing facilities and equipment, trained staff, good reporting systems, and so on. For many years Papua New Guinea did not have much of this when it came to HIV, and so the estimated prevalence has seen some dramatic shifts over time and has been a source of contention.

In 2001, when my colleagues and I were writing the grant proposal that would ultimately enable us to carry out comparative ethnography on married women's risk of HIV (Hirsch et al. 2010), there was almost no population-level HIV information for Papua New Guinea. In the absence of data, we represented Papua New Guinea as having a "nascent" epidemic, while the other countries in the study were categorized as either "concentrated" (that is, concentrated in highly vulnerable groups, such as sex workers) or "generalized" (that is, having spread from highly vulnerable groups to the general population). Within a few years, however, Papua New Guinea was categorized as having a generalized epidemic, apparently skipping the "concentrated" stage altogether. According to UNAIDS definitions, in a concentrated epidemic, HIV prevalence is less than 1 percent in the general population, but greater than 5 percent in at least one highly vulnerable group. In a generalized epidemic, HIV prevalence is greater than 1 percent in the general population. Women attending prenatal care clinics are typically used as indicators of "the general population." The few early epidemiological studies in Papua New Guinea showed a prevalence of 1.35 percent in women seeking prenatal care, and 17 percent in self-identified sex-workers in Port Moresby (WHO 2003, Mgone et al. 2002), which immediately put it in the "generalized" category. As worrying was that other research showed that women in rural areas had very high rates of multiple untreated sexually transmitted infections (Tiwara et al. 1996, Passey et al. 1998), a significant risk factor for HIV. This raised fears that if HIV moved into rural areas, it would spread extremely quickly—perhaps this was already happening, some policy makers said.

At the 2004 International AIDS conference in Bangkok, Papua New Guinea's minister for health, Melchior Pep, said "We're sitting under a devastating time bomb that is exploding as we speak" (Cullen 2006: 155). And Dr. Yves Renault, the World Health Organization representative in Papua New Guinea at the time, asserted that the "WHO estimates that two percent of PNG's population is HIV positive. . . . Our judgment is that, given the current level of infection and the rate of increase, it is possible that the number of infections could reach one million in 10–15 years unless decisive action is taken" (Cullen 2006: 155). Since Papua New Guinea's population at that time was six million, this was a frightening prediction. The 2006–10 National Strategic Plan on HIV/AIDS similarly asserted, "Papua New Guinea now faces a devastating HIV epidemic. If effective action is not taken, HIV will soon take a terrible toll on the people and the economy. It has been estimated that prevalence levels could reach about 18 per cent by the year 2010" (PNG NAC 2006: 14). Many of the factors that had shaped high prevalence in sub-Saharan

African countries were also found in Papua New Guinea: an economy dependent on mining and other extractive industries, high levels of untreated sexually transmitted infections, a highly mobile population, and acute gender inequality, including high levels of sexual and domestic violence.

However, these predictions of a catastrophic "African-style epidemic" (Cullen 2006) did not come to pass. Over time, based on more information from the rapidly increasing number of sites carrying out testing, estimates of HIV prevalence in Papua New Guinea have been continually adjusted downwards. In 2005, there were only 17 prenatal care HIV testing sites, but by 2013, this had increased to 329, multiplying the data for estimating HIV prevalence both nationally and by province. Globally, research showed that data from prenatal care clinics tend to overestimate population prevalence, and so the algorithm used to extrapolate prevalence from such data was changed, which also contributed to the downward adjustment of national prevalence in Papua New Guinea. Thus, the 2008 UN General Assembly Special Session (UNGASS) Country Progress report on AIDS in Papua New Guinea states: "The new estimated prevalence rate of 1.28 percent in 2006 among people aged 15–49, compared to the old estimates of 2 percent prevalence in 2005, does not represent in any way a decrease in the epidemic but the availability of better data and improved estimation methods" (UNGASS 2008: 11). And, in 2010, UNAIDS announced that "approximately 0.92 percent of the adult population in Papua New Guinea was living with HIV in 2009" (UNAIDS 2010). This estimated prevalence of .9 percent of the adult population remained true in 2016.

The changing epidemiological estimates necessarily altered the discursive representation of the epidemic, as well as national policy. For example, the 2014 Papua New Guinea Interim Global AIDS Response Progress & Universal Access Report asserts:

> Although it appears that PNG is now experiencing an epidemic concentrated in particular geographical locations and population groups, nearly all of our monitoring, evaluation and surveillance is still based on approaches more suited to a generalised epidemic. It is imperative that size & site estimations be conducted with men and women who sell and exchange sex and MSM in Port Moresby and other regional sites. (PNG NAC 2014: 16)

In other words, with the epidemic suddenly recategorized as urban and concentrated (rather than rural and generalized), there has been a significant shift in intervention strategies towards targeting MARPs (most at risk populations), also referred to as KAPs (key affected populations)—that is, female sex workers and men who have sex with men (MSM), particularly in urban areas and along major highways.

The profile of HIV in the Tari area appears to depart considerably from the current national narrative about the epidemic being concentrated in MARPs. Most of the thirty HIV-positive women I interviewed in 2011–13 had been infected by their husbands. They did not identify as sex workers, and most had not engaged in "transactional sex." In other words, they belonged to "the general population." Moreover, according to health workers at both clinics where I did research, most of the women registered with them were cases of husband-to-wife transmission. It is therefore important to keep in mind that one nation can contain multiple HIV epidemics, which may have different dynamics, even as they intersect with each other, and a national narrative may not capture a regional reality. The national .9 percent prevalence flattens and obscures significant variability across the country. I suspect that prevalence in Tari is significantly higher than the national average because of the nexus of factors discussed in chapters 1 through 3 that create HIV vulnerability: nearby resource-extraction projects, a period of severe economic decline and political abandonment, and high levels of marital conflict.

I came to suspect higher prevalence in the Tari area in part because five of the thirty women I interviewed had nuclear family members who were also HIV-positive: one's woman's brother had died of AIDS, another woman's brother was HIV-positive, one's woman's daughter was HIV-positive, one woman's sister had died of AIDS, and another woman's sister was HIV-positive. These family members did not have sexual partners in common (i.e., it was not the case that two sisters had sex with the same man), and in most cases they were living far apart from each other and thus not part of the same sexual networks. If prevalence was less than 1 percent, it seemed unlikely to me that a family would have more than one HIV-positive member. However, a sample of thirty is small, and there are, moreover, plausible social explanations for why HIV might cluster in some families. I remain concerned that the current national narrative does not capture the epidemiological reality of Tari, but I examine some of these family clusters and provide potential hypotheses for them in the first three chapters.

AIDS IN TARI'S POPULAR IMAGINATION

During Tari's most turbulent years, from the late 1990s to the mid 2000s, it became quite isolated, particularly in terms of services. The organizations that would normally have promoted AIDS awareness refused to send their staff there, fearing for their safety. Many local health workers fled, and those remaining felt abandoned and cut off from their normal institutional support. There was often no fuel, their vehicles broke down and couldn't be repaired, and in any case they were afraid to travel by road because of crime. So for a number of years, there was no formal AIDS education and no condom distribution. During this time, it was local churches that provided some information about HIV, though the pastors I spoke with said frankly that they had received no directions from their superiors about what they were supposed to tell their parishioners. The dominant ideas that circulated were highly moralistic: AIDS was described as a kind of divine punishment (Wardlow 2008; see also Eves 2003, 2012; Dundon 2007; Hammar 2010;

Kelly-Hanku et al. 2014), and those who died of AIDS-related illnesses were said to have brought this upon themselves through moral transgression, especially pre- and extramarital sex. When an AIDS patient's infant died, it was said to be part of the patient's punishment: the death would intensify his remorse for his sinful behavior and would work to erase his existence into the future. The fewer offspring he left behind, the fewer people there would be to carry on his lineage or remember his name. As one woman said to me, "God wants to exterminate the generations of people who might descend from the sinner. God wants to kill off his whole line so he will have no one to replace him on this earth. So his wife and child must die also. The smell of those sinners is offensive to God" (this was probably the most extreme statement I heard).

This is not to say that people did not know or understand that HIV was sexually transmitted—many people did. But when asked to describe how people became sick from AIDS, most resorted to a language of ultimate moral causality (divine punishment for sin), rather than proximate biomechanical causality (sexual transmission). Moreover, women were more often blamed for the spread of HIV than men. For example, the cause of AIDS was frequently attributed to women who "carry their genitals around and sell them [*karim tau raun na salim*]," a graphic way of describing sex work and transactional sex, and deliberately phrased to suggest an invidious comparison with women who carried around and sold other, appropriate goods, such as sweet potatoes.

By 2010, this morally condemning language had greatly diminished. ARVs had changed AIDS from a fatal disease to a potentially manageable one, making its conceptualization as divine punishment less compelling. Moreover, AIDS awareness initiatives had increased people's biomedical knowledge about modes of transmission, symptoms, and the availability of testing and treatment. People I spoke with in 2010–13 tended to know that the virus was found in blood and sexual fluids, that it was transmitted from one person to another through sex, that it wasn't transmitted through shared clothing or utensils, and that sharing razor blades was another possible means of transmission. HIV-positive people in treatment knew that sex with another HIV-positive person was not risk-free and could in fact have detrimental health consequences.

Such knowledge was often strongly inflected with Huli ideas about sex as a meeting of—or sometimes a confrontation or battle between—two bloods of differing strengths. Men are generally thought to have "stronger" blood than women, although the strength of a person's blood is not tied directly to gender. Rather, blood strength is tied to the force, energy, and charisma of one's persona: gregarious, extroverted, and assertive people have stronger blood. In the case of HIV, blood strength is said to affect the likelihood of transmission, as well as the activity of the virus: a person who is HIV-positive and has stronger blood is more likely to infect others, and a person who is HIV-negative and has stronger blood can "wake up" the dormant virus in a sexual partner who is HIV-positive and whose blood is weaker. Lucy, a widow ostracized by her siblings, said of her second husband:

> He had all these signs emerging on his body. He lost weight, he had diarrhea, he had sores on his skin. But I was fine. My body was fine, my blood was fine. But he was not all right. I thought it was my blood. I still think it was my blood. [You mean you think you infected him?] No, no. I think my blood hated his blood. My blood is strong, and so my blood kicked his blood. He had the virus, and he gave it to me, but my blood woke up his virus and made him sick.

Sex, more generally, was said to be a dangerous activity for HIV-positive people because of its heating properties: the heat of sexual activity could "wake up" and stimulate a virus, even if the virus was being "fenced in" by ARVs. These statements about battling bloods and sexual heat suggest that it is quite possible for people to possess basic public health knowledge about AIDS—for example, that HIV is found in blood and sexual fluids and can move from one person's body to another's through sex—without that knowledge mirroring a more mechanistic, depersonalized biomedical model. Moreover, such statements show that people are trying to make sense of the incomplete biomedical information they receive. They learn, for example, that HIV can live in the body for years without making a person noticeably sick, and this is translated during awareness talks as the virus "sleeping" in the body. It is not surprising, then, that people want to know what makes the virus "wake up." Similarly, people are told that ARVs "fence in" the virus or make the virus "sleep," again inviting questions about what might make the virus escape the fence or emerge from its torpor. People's solutions to the lacunae in the information they had received tended towards the moral, relational, and affective—they spoke of sexual heat, battling bloods, worry, and anger, issues I take up in chapter 5.

Men's and women's narratives about how they came to be infected also tended to be more complexly relational than standard global health messaging about modes of transmission. Anthropologists have often questioned public health messages' positing of a hyper-agentive autonomous actor capable of initiating and sustaining health-protective behaviors, regardless of socioeconomic context or relations of power. The counternarrative often proposed by anthropologists emphasizes the political, economic, and gendered structures of inequality that can make self-protective behaviors (e.g. condom use) impossible. In contrast to both of these models, the narratives related to me were often at a meso-level, between the individual and the structural, and assumed the causal primacy of the relational—most often family or kinship relations. HIV infection was sometimes ultimately attributed not to the infected person's own acts, or even to the infecting sexual partner, but to others' failures of care.

For example, one young man blamed his parents and his older siblings for his HIV-positive status. He had done well on the standardized test taken in grade nine—a huge hurdle, and one that dictates whether a student can go on to high school. However, his parents would not pay his school fees to continue. They had already invested in secondary and even tertiary education for some of his older siblings, and so they decided that they had enough educated and employed off-spring to take care of the rest of the family, and that he therefore did not need to pursue more education. He was so angry about this that he left Tari for the highlands city of Mount Hagen without any plans and found himself living in an informal urban settlement. Bitterly remembering this period, he said, "In the settlement, you know, everyone is just taking care of themselves. No one takes care of you." Lonely and struggling, he moved in with a woman there, and only much later learned that she was HIV-positive. He did not blame her for infecting him. Rather, he blamed his parents for not paying his school fees, and his older siblings for not sending him the money that might have put him on a less precarious path: "My life could have been like theirs, but no one in my family would care for me, so it is their fault that I got this virus."

Sometimes this relational notion of causality extended beyond persons to places, which were represented as exerting their own kinds of agentive influence over people. One older woman had been angrily separated from her husband for years, but when he came home during the 2002 election year as part of a poli-tician's entourage—well-dressed, ebullient, and handing out cash—she had sex with him. He was the person who had infected her—"I've never had sex with any-one else"—but she wasn't angry with him, for she also felt that Port Moresby, the nation's capital city, was to blame, and not because it was full of dangerous entice-ments that might lead men astray, but because returnees carried with them an aura of excitement, a kind of palpable charisma. She could feel it shimmering off of him as he descended from the plane, and she wanted to be part of it, so she agreed to have sex with him. The way she described it, she was less seduced by him than by the nation's capital, which he temporarily embodied.[5]

These examples of what might be called relational causality have a distinctively Melanesian feel to them. In Tari, individuals can, of course, be held solely respon-sible for their acts having injurious consequences for others or themselves, and yet there is also a willingness to recognize that a person's acts do not emerge only from the lone, interior self, but rather unfold from numerous prior social interac-tions and relationships. The Huli word for cause or origin is *tene*, which can also refer to tree roots, and just as the tree trunk emerges as a unitary form from a mostly unseen web of tangled roots, an event also emerges from a web of past interactions. Indeed, even persons might be said to appear to be unitary figures while actually being perpetually made and unmade by the gifts (e.g., school fees), substances (parental reproductive fluids), losses of personhood (from illnesses or being severely beaten), and nurturing or disciplinary acts by others. In the anthropological literature about Melanesia, this notion of the person is sometimes referred to as the "dividual" in order to distinguish it from Western/Northern assumptions about the bounded, singular, autonomous individual. As theorized by Marilyn Strathern, the dividual person is "constructed as the plural and composite site of the relationships that produced them" (Strathern 1988: 13). For the purposes of understanding how Huli often spoke about HIV infection—what I have called relational causality—the implications of dividual personhood are that there was often a presumption that other people played a part in creating the situation in which a person came to be HIV-positive. These narratives did not strip persons of intention, desire, agency, or responsibility, but rather acknowledged that their situations and actions were shaped by their past and present relations, and sometimes by the failures of others to care for them.

Huli people did, however, articulate a notion of ultimate causality regarding HIV infection beyond the relational. This was the idea that it was excess freedom—and especially the loss of custom as a protective moral "fence"—that had led to a multitude of social ills. "We are no longer fenced in" was a regular refrain, and AIDS was typically offered as proof of the problems caused by excess freedom. As it was explained to me, sociomoral rules, like fences, confine, but they also protect the self and others; they restrict, but they also enable moral development and flourishing. Describing yourself as having "jumped the fence" can be a way of saying that you are a rebellious, free spirit, but having "no one to fence you in" is also a way of saying that you have no one to care for you. Thus, when my interlocutors asserted that they were no longer fenced in as a people, they were decrying a loss of moral discipline, but they were also lamenting the sense of not being cared for (by the nation-state, for example).

The idiom of the fence to refer to moral discipline and care had multiple ramifications for HIV. For example, condoms, and sometimes even ARVs, were described as allowing people to "break the fence." The fear of being infected with HIV was said to be like a fence that prevented people from engaging in pre- or extramarital sex. Condoms, by allowing people to protect themselves from infection, and AIDS medications, by allowing people to recover from debilitating symptoms, broke the fence and tacitly gave people permission to behave in sexually transgressive ways with no repercussions. Some women I interviewed even spoke of HIV itself as a fence that forced them to behave in morally upright and constrained ways. Fear of infecting others, they said, made them careful about flirting with men or agreeing to spend time alone with them. And Lucy said that she used her ARVs to control her own movements: unlike many women who carried their medicine around with them, she deliberately left her supply at home so that she would have to return to take her evening dose and couldn't be tempted to stay out at night. As she plaintively put it, "I have no one to take care of me, no one to fence me in," and so she had to rely on her medication to assist her with this sociomoral work. Here we see that the relational and moral models of AIDS causality are intimately entwined: for women especially, kin have obligations of both discipline and care, and their failures leave women vulnerable to both moral waywardness and illness.

THE RESEARCH

This book is the culmination of two research projects, carried out over six periods of fieldwork between 2004 and 2013.[6] The first project, which entailed six months of fieldwork in 2004 and one month in 2006, was part of a multi-sited, comparative project investigating married women's risk of HIV in Papua New Guinea, Mexico, Nigeria, Uganda, and Vietnam (Hirsch et al. 2010). This research employed multiple methods, but at the center were semi-structured interviews with married men and women of different generations about their experiences of courtship, marriage, extramarital relationships, and mobility and migration, as well as their understanding of HIV/AIDS. For this research, I interviewed the female participants and trained four Huli male field assistants to interview the male participants, based on the assumption that men would be more candid about some topics, such as their extramarital liaisons, when speaking to another man. Each of my assistants completed at least ten interviews, so by the end of the research we had interviewed fifty-four married men and twenty-five married women.[7] A semi-structured interview guide, shared between all five field sites, was used for this research (see Hirsch et al. 2010, Appendix II), although it was adapted to each site. The interviews I did with women were done in Tok Pisin (Melanesian Pidgin) with Huli words and phrases thrown in when appropriate.

Tari proved to be a particularly challenging place to carry out the team's planned marital case-study methodology in which I was supposed to interview a married woman and a male field assistant would separately interview her husband. Huli men wanted to be interviewed first, and, once they knew the interview questions, many refused to give permission for their wives to participate in the research. Their objections included that wives might disparage husbands when interviewed, that talking about sex might arouse a wife and motivate her to be unfaithful, and that, as husbands who had given bridewealth for their wives, they were entitled to know how a wife had answered certain questions. I was loathe to make a woman's research participation contingent on male permission, but I ultimately concluded that interviewing the wife of a man who had already participated in the research but objected to her participation would entail far more risk of physical harm for her (through being punished by him) than she would encounter in her everyday life, and that there was little I could do to mitigate this risk. I was also concerned that her uncountenanced participation would be hazardous to me and my research assistants. Indeed, my field assistants were so distressed by the angry reaction of some of their peers to the request for their wives' participation that they informed me very early on in the research that they could not make such requests any more. In the end, we interviewed men and women who were married, but not to each other. This approach allowed individual women themselves to give or withhold informed consent and to hide their participation in the research from their husbands if they so chose. These interviews took place in a wide range of venues—at my guesthouse (I rented two rooms—one for myself, and one for interviews), in an empty trade store, in empty offices at the hospital, and in people's homes when they were alone. I came to know many of the women I interviewed quite well, because they would come back and visit, or I would run into them in town.

For the second project, carried out through fieldwork periods of six to ten weeks every year from 2010 to 2013, I investigated the lives of HIV-positive men and women who were in treatment. This research likewise entailed multiple methods, but primarily entailed clinic-based, semi-structured interviews with men and women (mostly women) about how they thought they had come to be HIV-positive, their decisions to seek testing and treatment, their experiences of disclosing their HIV-positive status to others, and their subsequent relations with friends, family, spouses and sexual partners, and community members. I rarely approached these women directly. Instead, clinic employees would inform women who had come to pick up their next three months' supply of ARVs that I was in a nearby room and interested in interviewing them if they were willing.

The women I interviewed were, on average, an older and less educated group than has been typical of much anthropological research about HIV: twenty of the thirty women fell roughly into the middle-aged and older category, and seventeen of them had no formal education or just a few years of primary school. Only one had completed high school. Thirteen of the women were widows (in every case their husbands had died of AIDS-related illnesses); ten were effectively divorced (they had either run away from or been abandoned by their husbands); three were currently married; and four had never married. The nature of this sample—and especially the average older age of the women—has some bearing on my findings, particularly women's reluctance to remarry, discussed in chapter 5. These interviews were also done in Tok Pisin with Huli words and phrases thrown in when appropriate.

The clinic-based interviews were limited in the sense that I only came to know those few women who lived near Tari town, and so never observed most of the participants in their households or communities. I did not visit any of the women who lived farther afield, in part because public transport was unpredictable, and in part because I did not want to draw undue attention to my research participants, even if many of them claimed that everyone in their community knew they were HIV-positive. I was able, however, to interview some of the women two or even three times, because the research took place over the course of four years. Thus, I learned how some of their situations changed quite dramatically from one year to the next.

AN OUTLINE OF THE CHAPTERS

I think of this book as having three parts. The first three chapters examine HIV vulnerability, and focus on the economic, political, and social factors that have produced some of the pathways through which women become infected. The last two chapters focus on women's experiences with their families and communities once they have entered treatment for HIV. And a chapter in the middle analyzes how the issue of gender is taken up in AIDS education workshops.

Chapter 1 examines the ways in which two resource-extraction projects near Tari, a gold mine and an oil-drilling operation, make women vulnerable to HIV. That mining towns are places of HIV risk is hardly a new finding. The social psychologist Catherine Campbell is perhaps best known among anthropologists for investigating and poignantly writing about the connections between migrant labor, the hazards of underground mining, masculinity, and men's relationships with sex workers at South African mines (Campbell 1997, 2000, 2003). In this chapter I argue that while Papua New Guinea's mining environment aligns with some of these findings, there are features of mining policy and practice in Papua New Guinea—in particular, "commuter mining" and the creation of a "landowner" class—that produce a unique kind of mine site and thus unique HIV vulnerabilities. For example, men who are designated as owners of the land leased to mining companies become wealthy and powerful patrons, and are able to demand fealty from their clients, including the "tribute" of wives. This has resulted in the trafficking of young rural women to mine sites, some of whom have become infected with HIV by their landowner husbands.

In chapter 2, I examine in greater depth the period of sociopolitical turmoil that Tari experienced from the late 1990s to the mid 2000s. This was the period in which many of the women I interviewed became infected, and I analyze these years as a time of abandonment by the state, characterized by flagrant crime, intensified warfare, the flight of public servants, and the evaporation of economic opportunities. I focus primarily on the increase in sexual violence during this period. Although my descriptions of sexual violence are not graphic, the reader should be warned that I closely examine cases of rape in which young women's accounts were questioned and they were publicly humiliated, resulting in suicide in one instance.

In chapter 3, I focus on gendered contestations over the meaning of marriage in Tari. A significant shift is taking place, with many younger people asserting the importance of marital choice and affective intimacy (Hirsch and Wardlow 2006). Nevertheless, men continue to aspire to polygyny as both a marker of and means to socioeconomic success. Thus, for many women, what began in youth as a companionate marriage founded in love and romance becomes a polygynous union in which they must sacrifice their own desires for intimacy, as well as the power that women can sometimes exert through being a man's sole partner. Often the emotional intimacy they had with their husbands was forged through years of shared strategizing and cooperative work devoted to getting ahead economically, making the material and affective dimensions of marriage deeply intertwined. When an additional wife comes into the marriage, often emotionally and physically displacing the first wife, the resulting bitterness and resentment play an important part in wives' decisions to engage in extramarital sex.

In chapter 4 I use a week-long AIDS education workshop as a case study for examining AIDS-awareness activities in Tari. Gendered inequalities, such as girls' and women's lesser access to education and employment, fuel the epidemic globally, and so AIDS awareness workshops often allocate a significant proportion of time to gender consciousness-raising, which typically includes discussions about gender stereotypes and gender-based violence. I analyze how the concept of gender was taught to the participants in this workshop, while also demonstrating that the workshop itself became a space where gendered tensions erupted and gendered inequalities were reproduced. AIDS educators must sometimes work hard to navigate and manage the gender inequalities and anger that emerge during AIDS-awareness activities, and this can spur "translational activism" (that is, the deliberate transformation or censoring of educational content) as they wrestle with material they find problematic.

Chapters 5 and 6 analyze the experiences of HIV-positive women who are on antiretroviral treatment. Chapter 5 discusses how women work to care for themselves; chapter 6 analyzes the steps they take to protect others and to demonstrate that they are ethical persons, not social threats. Chapter 5 focuses especially on the centrality of emotional regulation in women's self-care practices. Women living with HIV are counselled by health workers to avoid or "fence in" their negative feelings, such as anger and worry, which are said to "wake up" the virus or enable it to escape "the fence" that ARVs have built around it. Taking this advice to heart leads women to focus a great deal of attention on their inner lives, sensations, and feelings. For some women, fencing in their feelings entails physically fencing themselves within their own households, since they fear that once outside of the family property they might run into people who would cause them to feel anger. I draw on feminist theory about emotion and affect to analyze the potential epistemological and political consequences of controlling emotions that have been labeled dangerous.

Chapter 6, in contrast, discusses the moral quandaries that women encounter because of HIV stigma and their often economically reduced and socially contracted circumstances. Dependent on nuclear family members to take them in, and often considered morally suspect, some women take special pains to anticipate others' fears and to reassure them that they are the "safe" kind of AIDS patient, not the kind that would intentionally or carelessly infect others. They make a point of demonstrating to others that, as some women said, "I fence myself in [*mi banisim mi yet*]." Here, as mentioned earlier, the fence is a moral symbol of discipline and obedience to social expectations regarding proper female behavior. In this chapter I draw on feminist moral philosophy, especially Lisa Tessman's critical virtue ethics, to argue that HIV-positive women cultivate what Tessman calls "burdened virtues"—that is, virtues that enable a marginalized or oppressed person to manage their circumstances, but often at great cost to themselves.

The book as a whole provides a ten-year narrative about HIV in a place whose recent history has been turbulent and unpredictable, from the chaotic and desperate circumstances in which many women came to be infected to a period of relative plenitude characterized by good access to HIV testing, life-saving medicines, and medical care. It also highlights women's resilience, resolve, and humor in the face of vulnerability and violence.

1

"Rural Development Enclaves"

Commuter Mining, Landowners, and Trafficked Women

In 2000, I was in school, in grade four, and they came to get me, and I got married.[1] They came from Porgera. [And did you know him? Had you met him?] No, I didn't know him. His kin just came and got me. I didn't know what he was like, his living situation—I knew nothing about him. [So how did you come to marry him?] His kin just came and got me. They came to my family and described him to my parents and said to them, "Come get your bridewealth. It will be a lot." [So you didn't know him at all. How did he know about you?] Some of my kin were living in Porgera. He is a landowner, and they were living on his land. And he told them that he wanted a wife from them. And so my kin told him about me and said they would go get me for him. . . . And all they said to me was, "Oh, he's a wealthy landowner in Porgera. You'll live free. You'll have money. Oh, you'll live so well. You won't have to work in the fields. You'll eat lots of food from stores. You won't have to take care of pigs. Here in the bush you have to take care of pigs, and look at your hands and feet, covered with scars and callouses. If you marry this man you'll be able to sit down and rest. You'll live on money." It was all a con.

[Oh. So was it true what they had told you—that you would live on money and wouldn't have to plant sweet potato anymore?] No, it was all a con. There was a huge sweet potato field that I had to take care of all by myself. And another field that I used for growing extra produce that I sold. I worked really hard—I would get up early and go straight to the garden and work.

And my husband would sometimes follow me, sneak around in the ditches surrounding my gardens, and spy on me. He was jealous. He was always fucking around with other women, and this made him suspect that I might also be cheating. But I could always feel that someone was watching me, and a few times I caught him and I confronted him. I would yell out so anyone could hear, "Hey, why are you spying on me?! Are you my husband or are you some pervert criminal? Am I your wife or am I some young, unmarried girl that you are spying on?" So I shamed him for spying on me, and he would get angry that I'd caught him and was shaming him, and so a couple of times we fought in the field. The house too, we often fought at the house. [So you would hit him?]. Of course I did! I hit him. I whacked his legs with a spade. I cut his *arm with a knife. I hit him in the balls. He had to go to the hospital plenty of times because of me. I would yell, "What—you think I don't have hands?! You have hands to hit me? Well, I have hands too!" That's what I would say to him. He was always sleeping around with other women, but I didn't do anything wrong, and he would come and hit me. So I hit him back—I cut him. I would say, "I might have lost a lot of weight and look small, but I can still hit you and cut you. I'm the one who works in the garden every day—I have a lot of strength to beat you."*

[You had lost weight?] Oh, my sister (here Pamela shifted into the song-like register Huli women use to indicate sorrowful lament), my body didn't use to look like this, ohhh. My husband was always going around with out-side women, oh, ohhh. And my body changed completely, ohhh. I lost a lot of weight and I was sick all the time, oh, ohhh. (Shifting back to normal speech) And I wanted to go get a blood test at the hospital, but my husband said, "Why?" and he refused to go. And then I had a baby, and when it was four months old, it died. I took good care of it, but it died. So then I started to worry—this baby died, and I was sick all the time, and I developed lots of sores on my legs.

—PAMELA

I always asked the HIV-positive people I interviewed how they thought they had come to be infected, and resource extraction—gold, oil, and natural gas projects— was at the heart of the stories of eight of the thirty women. I return to Pamela later in this chapter, but here I want to highlight some significant themes in her narra- tive, because they point to the multiple pathways between resource extraction and HIV infection in Papua New Guinea. First is the figure of the "landowner"—or *papa bilong graun* (father/custodian of the land)—an identity category that has emerged from and become solidified by Papua New Guinea's resource-extraction policies and practices, particularly the need for mining companies to have social entities, represented by specific persons, with whom to negotiate and to whom to provide benefits, such as royalties or compensation for the loss of land (Jorgensen 2001; Golub 2007a, 2007b, 2014; Jacka 2015). The landowner is a potent and multi- valent symbol in the national imagination—landowners are envied, admired, and reviled. They are also economically and socially powerful people (almost always male) who can exert political influence, not only on their own communities, but also nationally or even internationally.

In Pamela's narrative, I would draw particular attention to the way that less powerful migrant Huli men attempt to overcome their "mining marginalization" (Jacka 2001: 46) by using women as a kind of tribute, cultivating or cementing ties to Porgeran landowners through marriage, a strategy that makes these women vulnerable to HIV. Pamela was her husband's third wife, so also important to note is the way that mining wealth is converted by landowners into additional wives and extramarital sexual liaisons (i.e., "outside women"), which not only exacerbates HIV vulnerability, but also generates marital distrust and suspicion that can erupt into violence. Finally, I would note women's determination, despite being structurally disadvantaged and vulnerable, to stand up for themselves both verbally and physically, a strongly socialized characteristic of Huli women (Wardlow 2006a).

In this chapter I analyze these resource-extraction sites—often referred to euphemistically in Papua New Guinea's HIV/AIDS policy literature as "rural development enclaves"—as spaces that produce HIV vulnerability. Some of the factors at play—a predominantly male workforce, the circulation of large amounts of cash, and the in-migration of women hoping to find transactional sexual partners—are not surprising and have been discussed in the rich literature about mining, migration, and HIV, particularly in South Africa (Campbell 2000; Crush et al. 2005, 2010). However, I argue additionally that the particular constellation of laws and policies that guide mineral and petroleum extraction in Papua New Guinea—such as "commuter mining" and the figure of the landowner—create a sexual economy that differs somewhat from the models of mining and HIV risk that are now canonical in the social science literature.

"NATURAL RESOURCE DEVELOPMENT ENCLAVES"

One might wonder what a "rural development enclave" is in Papua New Guinea. In the multi-million dollar Asian Development Bank (ADB) "HIV/AIDS Prevention and Control in Rural Development Enclaves Project," a rural development enclave is defined as "a particular area in a rural setting that has a significant private sector investment employing a relatively large number of people, has become a cash economy amongst a generally subsistence rural economy in the surrounding communities, and typically has become the major, or only, economic driver in the area" (ADB 2006a: 3). In other words, an enclave is defined geographically as a remote, rural site where a resource development project has created or massively intensified a cash economy and is, along with its affiliated subcontracting companies (e.g., trucking, janitorial, mess halls catering for employees), almost the only source of money in the area. Migration isn't specified in the ADB definition, but implicit is that a rural enclave is like a centripetal mass, with large numbers of cash- and opportunity-poor people moving to it from outlying areas. Porgera's population increased from approximately ten thousand in 1991, when the Porgera gold mine had just opened, to fifty thousand in 2010, almost all due to in-migration, Jerry Jacka estimates (2015: 185). Gender is also not explicitly mentioned in the above definition, but there are no "rural development enclaves" in Papua New Guinea where women make up the majority of the workforce or the primary recipients of other enclave benefits. Thus, also implicit in this definition is that most of the suddenly available money is in the hands of men, and many of the people drawn to these centripetal sites are women who, unable to gain access to the very few formal opportunities available to them, enter into various kinds of relationships with men to acquire cash.

"Enclave economies" are usually described by scholars as having high levels of formal employment (at least in comparison with surrounding rural areas, where there may be almost no employment) and high levels of foreign investment capital. What distinguishes a "resource-development enclave" economy from other kinds of foreign investment, however, is that value, in the form of the natural resource, is exported out the country, as are many of the skilled and foreign employees' wages. A defining feature of enclave economies is minimal integration with, or linkages to, the rest of the host country economy; thus, unlike other kinds of foreign investment, they may do little to sustain local industries or alleviate poverty (Gallagher and Zarsky 2007). Dependency theorists have therefore argued that enclave economies are damaging to underdeveloped countries, and while this view has been challenged, it is nevertheless the case that some mineral and petroleum companies have responded to such criticisms by trying to establish more linkages to local industries and businesses (Hansen 2014).

Another defining feature of enclave economies in Papua New Guinea is "commuter mining." Usually called FIFO—for "Fly-In, Fly-Out," because employees are typically transported in and out by plane or helicopter—commuter mining is a practice in which non-local employees (both foreign and Papua New Guinean) work very long shifts—typically twelve-hour days—every day for two to six weeks (the length varies enormously and depends on the company, the department, and the particular job), and are then transported for their breaks (also variable in length) back to their point of hire, which might be Cairns for Australian expatriate managerial employees, or cities like Mount Hagen or Port Moresby for non-local Papua New Guinean employees. FIFO has been a highly contested policy at some resource-extraction projects, not only in Papua New Guinea, but also in Australia, in part because it exacerbates the problem of minimal local economic linkages and business spinoffs (McGavin et al. 2001, Storey 2001, Filer and Imbun 2004, Connell 2005, McKenzie 2010). When Porgeran landowners were initially negotiating the Porgera Agreements—the documents signed by the national government, the Enga provincial government, and Porgera landowners that specify the benefits to be received by the community hosting the mine—they explicitly rejected the FIFO model. Instead they demanded the construction of a town in which employees would reside, and they imagined the establishment of an internationally and racially diverse mining community in which non-local staff would settle with their families for the duration of their contracts (Bonnell 1999; Jacka 2001, 2015).

There were both pragmatic and ideological impulses behind this demand. On the practical side, there was the expectation that the creation of a residential town would immensely benefit local construction businesses, that expatriate residents would spend their salaries on local goods, and that wealthier expatriate residents could demand infrastructural amenities that might benefit everyone, such as recreational facilities. Jerry Jacka (2015) describes an artist's rendering of this envisioned town as having a performing arts theater and a golf course. On the more ideological side, accompanying these expected business spin-offs was a vision of racial equality and concord: rather than white expatriates disappearing back to their well-appointed "real lives" elsewhere and treating Porgera as a remote, unknowable, and undesirable hardship post, expatriate employees would become locals who were invested in the community. "What seems very clear, from the way that local people talk about their foreign guests or tenants, is that they want nothing more (and nothing less) than a condition of equality and mutual respect between themselves and the expatriates who come to excavate their land," Colin Filer observes (2001: 15). The demand for a residential mining town is therefore not only about desired economic and infrastructural benefits. It is also an assertion about how expatriates (usually white) and Papua New Guinean citizens should live together, and it serves as an opening bid for trying to achieve this.

However, resource-extraction companies in Papua New Guinea generally resist demands that expatriate employees relocate, arguing that relocation will pose major recruiting and retention problems, since expatriate employees will avoid jobs that require their spouses and children to move to places that might put their safety in jeopardy and that do not have adequate educational, health, and recreational facilities. "Where social order remains volatile and opportunity costs of relocation are high, both employers and employees can be expected to seek to minimize physical and social contact with local communities," McGavin et al. comment (2001: 119); their surveys of non-national employees at eight different mines in Papua New Guinea showed 100 percent approval for FIFO in all but two of the sites (122). The Papua New Guinea Chamber of Mining and Petroleum, which represents the interests of these industries, has therefore consistently and vigorously argued in favor of FIFO. Thus, even in Porgera, where a relatively powerful group of landowners rejected FIFO, both from the outset and in its later negotiations with the mining company, all expatriate and most national employees nevertheless remain on FIFO contracts, and the town as envisioned was never built. Perhaps not surprisingly, the FIFO model is often perceived by local communities as a racist and/or classist rejection of rural Papua New Guineans. Many Huli now sardonically refer to their elected representatives as "FIFO politicians"—

that is, as urban elites who live in Port Moresby and only rarely fly in by helicopter to make a brief visit to their constituencies, much as FIFO expatriate mining employees only reluctantly, and in exchange for great compensation, agree to work at mine sites in Papua New Guinea.

The FIFO model creates enclaves with specific social and affective characteristics. For example, in order to compensate for the expense of constantly flying workers in and out of the country, FIFO employees work "compressed work schedules," as the literature euphemistically puts it. That is, as noted above, they work twelve-hour days for weeks at a time, leaving them exhausted and with little time or energy to establish feelings of connection to, or even interest in, the places where mines are located. When I stayed in Suyan, a residential compound of the Porgera Joint Venture (PJV) gold-mining operation, employees were up by 4 a.m. in order to have breakfast by 5, catch the shuttle to the mine site at 5:30, and begin work by 6. When they got off work at 6 p.m., they were in the mess hall by 7 for dinner, watched rugby on TV or used the gym for an hour, and were in bed by 9. The men I spoke with—mostly Australians, but some Papua New Guineans— knew next to nothing about Porgera and expressed no interest in learning about it. Far from the racially integrated community envisioned by landowners, for most non-local workers, Porgera is a place they have to go to in order to maintain their lifestyle at home.

Moreover, resource enclaves and their residential compounds for FIFO employees tend to be extremely securitized, with high razor-wire fencing, guarded gates, strict rules about whether and when employees may leave, and, in Porgera, a number of armed security forces on duty, including company security guards (443 of them in 2010, according to a Human Rights Watch report); the local Porgera police; "mobile squads," which are, as the name suggests, police units that are moved from place to place to deal with situations deemed urgent security matters; and Rapid Deployment Units, created in 1993 to protect national assets such as mines. These various security forces have mixed and shifting reputations: mobile squads, for example, are sometimes described as drunken, violent thugs. Intense securitization, arguably made more necessary by the lack of integration between the mine and the local community, contributes to HIV vulnerability. Police in general, and mobile squads in particular, regularly move from one posting to another, and they have a reputation for cultivating multiple sexual relationships wherever they are posted. Their mobility and multiple sexual partnerships, as well as the possibility that they coerce sex from female prisoners and from women who attempt to report rapes and assaults (Mcleod and Macintyre 2010), suggest that they are significant actors in Papua New Guinea's HIV epidemic, and this is likely intensified in places like Porgera, where there is a very large security contingent.

One woman I interviewed, Theresa, believed she had been infected with HIV by her Porgeran policeman husband, though she had had many other sexual partners after she left him, so the source of her infection is unclear. Theresa journeyed to Porgera when her brother Jethro was marrying his third wife, a woman from a Porgeran landowner family:

> We loaded lots and lots of bridewealth pigs into two trucks and drove them all the way to Porgera. And imagine!—I was a village girl. And when we were in Porgera we lived really well: we ate lots of store food and we rode everywhere in trucks. I saw people with lots of money—men with wads of kina shoved into their pockets. And I didn't want to go back—I wanted to stay. So when this policeman said he wanted to marry me, I said yes. [And were you his first wife?] No. He found women and left them, found them and left them. In fact, he already had a wife when I married him, but he didn't tell me this. He tricked me and said he wasn't married.

Probably for lack of additional housing, this policeman attempted to move Theresa in with his first wife, which did not go well:

> I arrived, and his first wife stabbed me with a knife. And I stabbed her back, in the neck. [Did she die?] No (laughing). I injured her, but I didn't kill her. She stabbed me when my back was turned, but I turned around and grabbed her knife and poked her in the neck. It was good that I did that, because I really scared her. She was afraid that I would kill her, and so she ran away. Then the house was mine. I lived there for five years.

Most Huli women are taught and encouraged by their mothers, sisters, and other female kin to be physically assertive and to respond to physical aggression, especially from other women, with equal or escalated aggression (Wardlow 2006a). In this case, the first wife's attempt to intimidate Theresa backfired, and she ended up making a hasty retreat, leaving Theresa with dominion over the house. Ultimately, however, Teresa left:

> When I lived with him, he would often leave and be gone for a while, and sleep with lots of other women, and he made me sick lots of times. [Do you mean sick with gonorrhea, that kind of illness?] Gonorrhea, other sicknesses, I don't know. I think he infected me with this virus.

Also contributing to the role that intensive securitization can play in creating an HIV risk milieu is the fraught relationship between local residents and security forces. PJV security personnel have shot illegal miners caught inside the mine site, for example, and local communities often retaliate when this happens, which can lead to a vicious cycle of escalating violence. Included in my interviews is a narrative by a Huli woman who said she and a friend had aided a local gang in assaulting two Porgera policemen and stealing their guns: they told the officers that they had missed the last bus home to their village and begged them for a ride, saying they were afraid to walk home after dark. They then lured them into a car-jacking. Moreover, it is now internationally known that PJV security personnel raped Porgeran women who had been caught trespassing and looking for gold on PJV's waste rock dumps. According to the Human Rights Watch report about these abuses, a factor that contributed to the guards' violence was their fear of and anger about violent daily raids on the mine by groups of illegal miners (Human Rights Watch 2011). Thus, as an affective environment, one might characterize the PJV enclave as immersed in fear, anger, and distrust.

SITUATING TARI AMONG THE SURROUNDING ENCLAVES

The Tari area is not itself a "rural development enclave," but it is located between three major resource-extraction sites, and residents thus can be considered a satellite population of all of them: an oil-drilling project operated by Oil Search Ltd., with a large base in Moro, Southern Highlands Province; the Porgera Joint Venture gold mine, just over the border in Enga Province, north of Hela; and, most recently, ExxonMobil's PNG LNG, based in Hides, not far from Tari, which was in the construction phase during the final years of my research in 2010–13.

For the resource projects based in Hela Province, Huli receive some benefits, such as preferential hiring, and many Huli men are employed either by the companies themselves or by landowner companies contracted to do specific jobs, such as transport or janitorial services. In contrast, Huli do not receive direct benefits from the PJV gold mine, but many Huli have long-standing ties of ritual, trade, and intermarriage with Ipili people in Enga Province who do receive benefits, and it is these kinds of ties and claims—and not employment at the mine—that bring them to Porgera. Indeed, the few Huli men I knew who had attempted to get jobs with PJV said that they were expected to pay exorbitant bribes in order to be put forward by the hiring committee, controlled by Porgera landowners (see also Jacka 2001: 49). Thus, many Huli migrate to Porgera hoping for economic opportunities—searching for gold in the mine's waste rock; engaging in artisanal mining; or simply becoming a kind of hanger-on, waiting for economic possibilities to emerge. Having sketched out some general characteristics of "resource development enclaves," I turn to a discussion of how Moro and Porgera have shaped HIV risk for people residing in the Tari area, especially women.

Oil Search and Moro

The impact of Oil Search's oil-extraction activities is not immediately felt in Tari, because there is no direct road between Tari and Moro, where Oil Search's drilling operations are based. Oil Search's employees therefore tend to travel to other towns, such as Mendi or Mt. Hagen, to spend their wages. However, even if Oil Search's presence in Tari is not easily felt or seen through its employees' consumption patterns, it has shaped Tari as an HIV risk milieu: three of the thirty women I interviewed who were on ART had been infected by husbands who worked at Moro, two as employees of Oil Search, and one for a landowner company contracted by Oil Search.

More than many other resource-extraction companies in Papua New Guinea, Oil Search has a reputation for a strong commitment to corporate social responsibility and to addressing health issues, not just for its employees, but also for the communities surrounding its projects. And, compared to ExxonMobil, for example, Oil Search has a far more savvy and astute sensibility regarding community relations, aware that spreading services and goodwill widely, even far beyond the official boundaries of its project sites, is worth the expense for the community support it garners. In the Tari area, for example, Oil Search employees will sometimes give rides to older women carrying heavy loads of sweet potatoes from their gardens (a practice that violates the rule against non-employees in their vehicles), and although they refuse to give in to the young men who sometimes block roads and demand payment to pass, they will nevertheless give those same young men cash on other occasions (that is, as gifts, not extortion) or hire them for community projects, such as cleaning up roadside trash.

Another indication of Oil Search's commitment to social issues is that when it was determined that neither the Papua New Guinea Department of Health nor NGOs in the country had the technical capacity to manage grants from the Global Fund to Fight AIDS, Tuberculosis and Malaria, Oil Search created the Oil Search Health Foundation and formally became the principal recipient for the country, in charge of disbursing funds to, and monitoring and evaluating the projects of the implementing sub-recipient organizations, such as Save the Children. Doubtless there was self-interest involved in this step (i.e., access to Global Fund money for health and development projects in the communities where Oil Search extracts resources); nevertheless, this proved to be an extremely challenging and onerous undertaking: I was told by one expatriate Oil Search Health Foundation employee that the monitoring and reporting requirements for the Global Fund were more elaborate, time-consuming, stressful, and unrealistic than those of any oil company or NGO he had ever worked for.

Another example of Oil Search's commitment to corporate social responsibility has been its willingness to collaborate in HIV/AIDS research by the Papua New Guinea Institute of Medical Research (IMR) and the Papua New Guinea National Research Institute (NRI). Its cooperation in these endeavors means that there is a relatively large amount of data regarding employees' behaviors and practices, more than is readily available for other mine sites. One piece of research by NRI (Buchanan et al. 2011), for example, investigated employees' alcohol consumption, sexual behavior, condom use, and knowledge about HIV. It showed that the nature of Oil Search employment contracts—particularly the very long tours of duty entailed by the FIFO model—contributed to HIV vulnerability by shaping employees' sexual behavior, both on-duty and off. Based on interviews with over four hundred employees, the research team found that "three main patterns for breaks were evident when workers were asked how many days they worked before

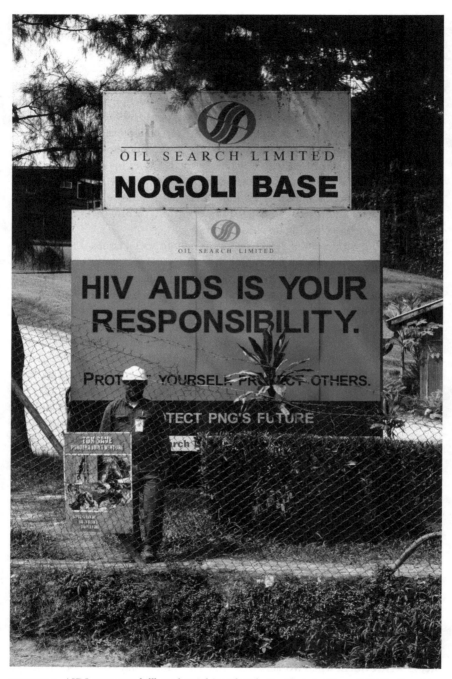

FIGURE 3. AIDS awareness billboard at Oil Search Ltd. site. Photo by Kenneth I. MacDonald.

they went on break: 39.0 percent took a break after four weeks (28 days) and close to half (48.2 percent) reported having breaks after six weeks (42 days)" (Buchanan et al. 2011: 43). Given long workdays, company guidelines prohibiting sexual relations between co-workers, and rules against leaving the residential compounds at night, it is not surprising that 82 percent of all employees said they did not have sex when on duty. Many of the employees lamented that the long tours of duty were damaging to their relationships at home and made them hunger for sex. In contrast, when off duty, the exchange of sex that happens outside the camp area was accepted by workers as normal. During time off, men spent time with people in the community, including in clubs where there is contact with women exchanging sex for money and other goods. There was also *dinau koap* (literally, debt sex), an arrangement where men would have sex with sex workers on credit and the women could come to the gates on pay days to be paid (Buchanan et al. 2011: 66).

Of those employees with FIFO arrangements, nearly half of the male employees who transited through large urban centers, particularly when coming off duty, had paid for sex when transiting (Buchanan et al. 2011: 46). Approximately 25 percent of the male employees had paid for sex in the past year. A third of these men reported inconsistent condom use, and 15.5 percent reported that they had not used a condom with any sexual partners during the previous three months (Buchanan et al. 2011: 71). It would appear, then, that the FIFO model of labor contributes to the production of a particular kind of sexual economy in which workers must largely abstain from sex during the four to six weeks that they are on duty, but then freely engage in a range of transactional sexual relationships when off duty, both in the nearby community and in the urban areas through which they transit.

As noted above, three of the women I interviewed had been infected with HIV by husbands employed at Moro. One of these women, Kori, had dropped out of school after grade 4 because her parents wouldn't pay her school fees, and she spoke with resentment about the fact that they had been willing to pay for her two younger brothers, both of whom had made it through high school and beyond. Without an education, her means of making money became the same as most uneducated rural women in Papua New Guinea: selling betel nut by the side of the road. It was while doing this that she met her husband. He was driving a company vehicle, stopped to buy some betel nut, and flirted with her. He continued to do this for a few weeks, and each time they talked a little more. Although she felt too young to marry, she also felt lucky to have gained the attentions of a well-paid "company boy," as Huli people sometimes call them, and so she agreed to marry him.

Although he initially always came home when his month-long shift ended, he began staying in the Moro area during his breaks when she became pregnant, and gradually he came home less and less. She heard gossip that he had other sexual partners, but she said nothing because he was a generous and reliable provider. It was when she heard that he had a relationship with a woman rumored to be HIV-positive that she insisted that they get tested: "And I told him, 'If you've given it to me, I want to die on my own clan land. If I die, I die, but I'm not staying with you.' [What did he say?] What could he say? There was nothing to say. I told him I was leaving, and when we tested positive, I left."

It would be incorrect, however, to think of all "company boy" wives as put in the path of HIV by their own desires to move beyond their less privileged backgrounds or the educational disadvantages they faced because they were girls. Another woman, Jody, whose father and two brothers worked at Moro, had completed high school and done one year of business college when she met the man who was to become her husband, also an employee at Moro. From her own observations and from talking to her brothers, she "knew what company boys were like" and how they behaved when on break—that is, she knew their reputation for having many sexual partners. But, she was in love, and so "I closed my eyes and married him (*mi pasim ai na go marit*)." In other words, she knew the possible risks, but chose to ignore them and hoped for the best. "Later I found out that he had slept around with a lot of women before we married and continued to do so after we were married. But, it was hard for me to leave him. When I learned he was fucking around (*guap guap raun*), I tried, but he came after me and brought me back."

In 2006, her father, who had driven to Mendi Hospital to pick up supplies for the Moro health center, observed her husband in the area where HIV tests are done. HIV testing is available at Moro, so Jody's father was made suspicious by the fact that her husband chose to be tested in Mendi. To his mind, this meant that her husband probably suspected he was HIV-positive and wanted to minimize the possibility of others finding out by getting tested elsewhere, a common strategy, especially for men, since they are more mobile than women. He informed Jody about what he had seen and advised her to leave her husband. Soon after, her husband left for Port Moresby without telling her, so she was unable to confront him about his HIV test. In 2007, when testing became widely available in Tari, she herself went for testing and was found to be positive. She did not begin treatment until 2008, when her symptoms of diarrhea, fevers, and weight loss were becoming severe. Her husband died in Port Moresby in 2008, and she believed that he never sought treatment, despite easy availability in the capital city, probably because of shame. Men's failure to be tested, or their tendency to seek testing and treatment far too late, was a story I heard repeatedly.

That shame or fear thwarted HIV testing and treatment was not confined to men, of course. Jody's own younger sister, whose husband worked for a resource-extraction company other than Oil Search, had died of AIDS-related illnesses in 2011. Despite knowing that Jody was HIV-positive and successfully on treatment, her sister could never bring herself to come to terms with her diagnosis:

> Her husband would come and go to Port Moresby, but spent most of the time in Port Moresby. And she lost weight, but at first we just thought she missed him or was worried about him or was lonely. We didn't think she was sick. But then she kept losing weight, a lot of weight. And so I told her, "Your husband lives far away

and we don't know how he behaves when he's not here. You should get a blood test." [So you suspected?] Yes. So I came with her to get a blood test, and she was positive. . . . .

[So when you knew you were both HIV-positive, did you live together and take ARVs together?] No, she was living in T—, and I was in H—. And she only started taking ARVs when she got very, very sick. The medicine didn't work for her. I think she was already full of the virus when she started taking ARVs. And the virus must have infected her brain because she became very confused, and then she stopped making any sense at all (*toktok bilong em go kranki olgeta*). . . . .

She died in 2011. I miss her lot—she always took care of me when I was sick, she always listened to my worries, she was like my second mother. [Did her death make you afraid or worried, since you are also HIV-positive?] No, it just made me very sorrowful, because I have this illness, so I know what it is like, and I believe that if she had started taking this medicine earlier she would still be alive. I told her and told her to go to the hospital, but she gave up and wouldn't go. [Why did she give up?]. She was supposed to go back after the blood test and get her results, but she wouldn't go. I was the one who went and found out her results. They were willing to tell me because they knew I was HIV-positive and that I was her sister and could help her. They had told her to come back in two weeks for the results, but she refused. I think she just didn't want to know, she was afraid, and so she delayed and delayed. And then it was too late.

Although we'll never know what Jody's sister was thinking or feeling, her case suggests the powerful role that the fear of death and stigma can play, even when a woman has strong family support and evidence within her own family of ART's efficacy.

This case is also one of the nuclear family clusters of HIV that I discussed in the Introduction. These family clusters made me skeptical about the supposed low prevalence of HIV in Papua New Guinea, or at least made me suspect that some areas of the country, like Tari, have a prevalence far higher than the national average. Is it likely, I asked myself, that I would have found so many cases of HIV within nuclear families if prevalence was truly .9 percent? And yet this is a case in which a plausible explanation based on social dynamics might help to explain such family clusters without resorting to the conclusion that HIV prevalence must be high in the Tari area. Having been raised in a family where all the men worked for resource-extraction companies, and having become accustomed to a relatively higher standard of living, it is hardly surprising that both Jody and her sister chose to marry men who also worked in that industry. Born into a relatively wealthy rural class, they both strove to retain and consolidate that class through marriage. Though they knew that male employees were reputed to have many sexual partners, they did not know that their class-retention strategies were putting them at relatively greater risk of HIV infection.

PJV and Porgera

Porgera Joint Venture (PJV), one of the top-producing gold mines in the world, is located in Porgera, Enga Province, just over the border from Hela Province.[2] The

Asian Development Bank proposal cited earlier notes that while average national HIV prevalence was estimated to be 2 percent in urban areas and 1 percent in rural areas, "Out of 920 persons tested at Porgera Hospital in 2004, 7.7 percent were infected with HIV" (ADB 2006b: 3). Notably, while HIV prevalence among PJV employees was approximately the same as national prevalence (2 percent), it was much higher—8 to 10 percent—in the rest of the Porgera community (Corporate Social Responsibility Newswire 2007). When I spoke to PJV medical staff in 2006, they expressed puzzlement and alarm at this large discrepancy. However, some of the specificities of Porgera as a mine site help to explain why HIV prevalence has been so much higher in the Porgera community than among PJV employees.

Much of the social science literature on mining and HIV vulnerability focuses on the mine worker—the usually male person who, while often sacrificing his well-being for his family, ends up infecting wives and girlfriends with STIs and HIV. Catherine Campbell's research with black South African miners highlighted the exhausting work, the gnawing fear of death deep underground, and the long absences from home that provoked fatalism, loneliness, and the desire for comfort and the sensation of being viscerally alive, for example—feelings that the miners tried to manage through drinking and sex (1997). That mining labor is predominantly male, and mine culture often highly masculinist, also contribute to regular binge drinking and unprotected sex. The literature seeking to quantify the beneficial impact of family housing on HIV risk is scant (Gebrekristos et al. 2005), but in addition to these factors, some researchers blame mining companies' failure to provide family housing for employees, which might help to curb the high levels of extramarital sex resulting from miners' long absences from home.

The Porgera mine site is characterized by a number of these factors. The work force is mostly male (in 2010, 8 percent of PJV's staff—196 out of 2,408—were women); alcohol is readily available (although its importation into and sale in Enga Province are prohibited); and many women have migrated to the area for sex work (PEAK 2011). There are, however, significant differences between South African mines and Porgera, and these differences demonstrate the importance of taking into account factors like national mining policies, the nature of employee contracts, and the housing of employees in analyzing HIV vulnerability at resource-extraction sites. For one thing, the housing of PJV employees would appear to be markedly unlike the situations described by Catherine Campbell (2003), Dinah Rajak (2011), and Donald Donham (2011), all of whom discuss mining employees coming and going freely from men-only residences, with some employees opting to live in the adjacent townships rather than in the mine's hostels. In contrast, non-local PJV employees live in highly securitized compounds, and their movements tend to be only by vehicle and only to travel back and forth to the mine site for work, while local employees (i.e., Porgerans) commute from their villages or live with town-dwelling kin.

Occupational safety would seem to be another difference. PJV has an excellent occupational safety record, and underground mines in Papua New Guinea are not anywhere near as deep as those in South Africa. PJV miners are therefore not subjected to the claustrophobic and dread-inspiring caged mine shaft elevators described by Campbell's (1997) and Donham's (2011) informants. While some PJV miners work underground, the mines are shallow enough that they can be driven to their work sites. During my two brief visits to Porgera to discuss HIV prevention strategies with PJV managers, there was a large billboard as one entered the mine site that informed everyone how many "injury free days" had passed, and all the departments I visited began their day with a meeting in which the discussion of occupational safety seemed to be accorded almost as much time as the presentations on how much ore had been excavated and how much gold processed the previous day. In other words, mine safety ranked very high in importance. This is all to say that PJV miners probably do not experience the existential terror and fatalism Campbell describes as playing an important part in motiving South African miners' sexual relationships.

On the contrary, it is likely that fear plays a part in *deterring* non-local employees from having sexual relationships with local women. Owing to ongoing tensions and episodic violent hostilities between the mine and the local community, between different landowning groups, and between landowner and non-landowner groups, PJV'S residential compounds are guarded by armed security personnel and surrounded by high fences topped with razor wire. The buses that transport employees from their fenced residential compounds to the mine and back have thick metal mesh on the windows because of past incidents when local residents threw stones at them. Jacka documents increasing violent conflict in the Porgera area, largely between those who receive benefits from the mine and those who do not, claiming that "for many of the young men in Porgera . . . warfare is the new economy" (2015: 224), with clans buying black-market M16 assault rifles and hiring out their young men as warriors to other clans. It is therefore likely that the strict security procedures, the fear of violence in Porgera, the PJV policy that forbids alcohol consumption, and the FIFO policy of extremely long hours, followed by mandatory breaks away from Porgera, all combine to prevent non-local employees from having sexual liaisons during their rostered twenty days on. Moreover, information about AIDS has been readily available to PJV employees since at least 2004, as have condoms: when I visited in 2004 and 2006, free condom dispensers were everywhere at the mine: the airport terminal, offices, break rooms, bathrooms, and so on.

Local employees, in contrast, may very well be engaging in a range of sexual relationships with multiple partners in Porgera. But, again unlike the black miners in South Africa, they are not migrants, they are not estranged from their families for months at a time, and many have wives and children to return to when their shifts are over. In sum, the way that PJV mining labor is organized

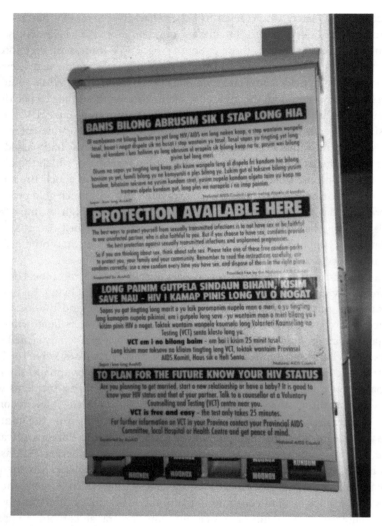

FIGURE 4. Free condom dispenser at Porgera Joint Venture mine site. Photo by author.

and disciplined, both spatially and temporally, means that the sexual economy in Porgera, and how miners are able to engage with it, differs significantly from that in South Africa described by Campbell and other scholars. And given the constraints on PJV employees' mobility within Porgera, perhaps it should not be surprising that HIV rates among PJV employees are roughly the same as the national urban average.

The case with the rest of the Porgera community is another story, and the Porgeran landowner plays an important role in it.

PORGERAN LANDOWNERS

Joshua Barker and his colleagues employed a novel way of analyzing the social fabric of modernity in Southeast Asia through the trope of "the figure," which they described as "persons within a given social formation whom others recognize as symbolizing modern life" (2013: 1)—for example, a photo retoucher in Vietnam or a timber entrepreneur in Malaysia. Providing rich portraits of eighty such figures in nine countries, they note that "Just as the *flaneur* makes sense only against the backdrop of emerging mass commodification in nineteenth-century Paris, so too do the figures in this volume make sense only once they have been set against particular backgrounds" (4). They quote Ara Wilson (2004: 191), who asserts that "capitalist development comes with its own figures, personae that represent new modes of work and new styles of being," persons who are "embodied symbols of the promise and problems of new economic realities." In any analogous compendium of "figures of modernity" in Papua New Guinea, the landowner would surely be at the top of the list.

The landowner is the feature of Porgera that most differentiates it from the South African mines discussed by Campbell, Rajak, and other social scientists. And, as shown by Pamela's story that began this chapter, the impact of landowners stretches beyond Porgera and into populations on its margins, such as Tari. The landowner is a person who can make demands and wrest things from government elites and multinational corporations in ways no one else can, and who embodies the promise of "development," or perhaps even the possibility of bypassing "development" (in its implicit sense of only gradual improvement) in achieving swift and dramatic prosperity and power. The landowner also embodies the problems of Papua New Guinea's economic dependency on mining. As Jacka notes,

> Expensive cars, new clothes, luxury food items, and partying trips to Mt. Hagen constitute the bulk of SML [special mining lease] landowners' purchases. Porgera has also seen key players within the SML landowning clans becoming big men on a far larger scale than customary political economics allowed. Many of these men spend their days driving around the government station at Porgera in new model Toyota Land Cruisers with dark-tinted windows; nearly all are polygynists, some with as many as twelve wives. (2015: 210)

All land in Papua New Guinea not appropriated by the government prior to passage of the Land Act of 1962 is legally held by customary landowning groups, although subsoil resources are owned by the state. Since 97 percent of PNG's territory had not been appropriated, one might assume that almost all Papua New Guinea citizens must be landowners; however, with the extractive industry accounting for approximately 70 percent of the country's export earnings, the term "landowner" has come to refer only to those people—and typically only the men—whose land sits atop natural resources that a company plans to excavate. In order to develop a mine, a mining company must take out a "special mining lease" (SML) in which it is the tenant, and the customary inhabitants thereby become landlords of sorts who have the right to compensation for the loss of their land. In other words, national law "requires the existence of a formally recognized group of 'native landowners'" (Golub 2007: 39) who normally gain this legal recognition by forming Incorporated Lands Groups (ILGs).

Victoria Stead notes that it is through these ILGs that communities "*become landowners* in a way that is 'legible' (Scott 1998) to the sites and agents of the state and globalizing capital" (2017: 364, emphasis in original). In other words, ILGs provide corporations and government departments something to interact and negotiate with. However, she adds, "Doing so involves not simply a translation, but a transformation of the nature of connection to land" (2017: 364). Specifically, inhabitants' connection to land becomes defined as a property relation. As Filer et al. explain this transformation, "Land is separated from human labour, local livelihoods and personal relationships, and made into a substance that can be mapped and surveyed, quantified and measured, divided and subdivided, without any necessary reference to its cultural and natural attributes" (Filer et al. 2017: 18). And, of course, for landowners, it becomes a substance that they relinquish and see transformed, or even destroyed, in exchange for money and other benefits. Filer et al. argue that if inhabitants willingly, or even enthusiastically, form ILGs in order to negotiate with resource companies, "it is not because they favour the accumulation of capital at their own expense, but because they believe (rightly or wrongly) that 'developers' will provide them with rental incomes, business opportunities, or even some of the public goods and services, from roads to scholarships, that cannot be obtained from their governments" (2017: 30).

Before mining leases are issued, a benefits-sharing agreement must be reached with landowners, and, in the case of the Porgera mine, this includes royalty checks every three months, monetary compensation for the loss of land and houses, preferential hiring at the mine, preference for contracts with the mine, and relocation housing. One study of PJV mining benefits from 1990 to 2009—which included royalties, wages, taxes, compensation payments, and contracts—found that the national government received K1.7 billion while Porgeran landowners received almost as much at K1.2 billion (Johnson 2010). In other words, many of the benefits from resource extraction are intensely localized, and one aspect of the "ideology of landownership" (Filer 2001: 9) is "the pervasive view at the popular, grassroots level that benefits from mining *should* be local rather than national" (Filer and Macintyre 2006: 219; emphasis added).

The policy of preferential benefits to landowners is deliberate: it is intended to secure the ongoing consent of landowners to the extraction of wealth from their land. However, the policy creates massive discrepancies between those who happen to reside on land that rests atop gold and their neighbors and kin who do not. As Victoria Stead notes, "Practices of land formalisation are exercises in boundary making, and this is a key way in which they function to exclude. Incorporated land groups make landowners, in effect, by drawing boundaries around them. They provide a mechanism for determining who is and is not a recognised right-holder" (2107: 364–65). Consequently, as Jerry Jacka vividly describes it, "At the Porgera Station market, landowners drive up in their new Toyota Land Cruisers and saunter around the stalls in their latest fashions listening to their headphones or playing a hand-held video game. Meanwhile, their non-landowner kin sit beside a pile of vegetables for sale, barefoot and wearing second-hand clothing, hoping they will make enough money to at least pay for the PMV ride back to their own village" (2001: 50).[3]

The stakes for being designated a landowner are obviously quite high. And, in many regions of Papua New Guinea, the identification of stable and pre-existing entities that might be termed clans or landowning groups has been a formidable task that has entailed some willful invention, or at least vigorous transformation, of indigenous sociality. For instance, all the ethnographers who have done research in Porgera assert that, as Alex Golub puts it, "Porgeran kinship is less a matter of corporate groups than of a large mesh of egocentric personal networks" (2007a: 83; see also Biersack 1995, Golub 2014, Jacka 2015). Much like the Huli, Porgerans assert that they descend from the ancestors of both their parents and can thus claim membership in eight clans (their FFF's clan, their FFM's clan, their MFF's clan, their MFM's clan, and so on). Membership depends on genealogical ties, but also upon activating and maintaining those ties through agricultural labor, commensality, visiting, and contributing to bridewealth, warfare, and homicide compensation payments. Few people can actually say they are members of eight clans, though many claim four or five. Moreover, Porgerans (and Huli) "do not consider it a virtue to identify strongly with only one clan" (Golub 2014: 124); rather, they seek multiple affiliations. And "clans"—although this should be considered an expedient term that has reifying effects which misrepresent Porgeran sociality—do not, in fact, act corporately: clan members do not pay bridewealth together or even necessarily make war together. As Jacka notes, and this would be true of the Huli as well, "Linguistically it may appear as though it is the activities of one clan that is engaging in these events, such as when people say that Tokoyela fought Undiki, or Tokoyela made a compensation to Pakoa. In reality one group of people from multiple clans is engaging with another, similar group" (Jacka 2015: 124). Rather than acting as corporate entities, then, individuals mobilize their "cognatic portfolios" (Golub 2014: 150) in times of need.

Eliciting, reifying, and delimiting bounded formal groups from this flexible array for the purposes of negotiating mining agreements and allocating mining benefits has been challenging at best and deadly at worst. In the Porgeran case, it was determined that seven Ipili "clans," comprised of twenty-three "subclans," were the official landowners within the PJV SML, and each subclan appointed a member to the Landowner Negotiating Committee. However, as Golub notes, "it was not so much that twenty-three subclans had representatives as that twenty-three important people had 'solidified' . . . twenty-three subclans that they could represent" (2014: 97–98). Moreover, many of the Porgeran landowners belong to multiple subclans and thus receive multiple royalty checks, and landowners often try to marry strategically by taking wives from additional subclans in order to secure additional benefits.

Much of the anthropological work on Papua New Guinean landowners has, perhaps not surprisingly, focused on the landowner as an elicited and even invented category—that is, a category of person that has emerged in response to the requirement that resource-extraction companies and the state interact with them (Golub 2014, Ernst 1999, Jorgensen 2001, Gilberthorpe 2007). Less attention has been paid to the kind of personhood that landowners enact or embody. Landowner groups, perhaps especially Highlander landowner groups, are often vilified by mining company personnel (at least behind closed doors) for their negotiating tactics: they are said to hold projects hostage until demands are met, renege on agreements, attempt to extract more benefits after agreements have been finalized, demand financial compensation for injuries that seemingly have little to do with a project's impact, and so on (Filer 1998, Golub 2007b). Indeed, one survey of mining and petroleum companies in Papua New Guinea identified landowners as the number one issue negatively affecting the resource-extraction industry (Imbun 2006). Moreover, particularly in the wake of ExxonMobil's LNG project, which during its construction phase bestowed immense sums of money on Huli landowners, landowners have become associated with excessive, wasteful, arrogant, drunken, promiscuous, and sometimes bullying and boorish behavior, not only in their places of residence, but also in Port Moresby's hotels and bars.[4]

People are often afraid of landowners. When non-local Papua New Guinean PJV employees drove me around the Porgera area, I observed that they always recognized and gave way to landowner vehicles when encountering them on one-lane roads and bridges, not wanting to risk the possibility that a landowner might feel disrespected and be motivated to retaliate in some way. And, although PJV employees were supposed to report even minor incidents of conflict with the local community (e.g., when a drunk person swore at them or threw a stone at a PJV vehicle), they did not always do so when landowners were involved.

It is important to note that there are wide discrepancies in wealth, not only between landowners and non-landowners, but between landowners. For example, the twenty-three Porgeran landowner subclans do not all receive the same amount in royalties because these depend on the amount of land a subclan owns within the SML; some subclans own a lot and some very little.[5] So, as Jacka observes, "At one extreme are the SML 'super big men' with their multiple wives, business holdings, and new cars" (2015: 210); then there are the landowners whose subclans own very little land within the SML; and then there are the people who are landowners within "the project area"—that is, they do not belong to the twenty-three subclans who own land within the SML, and thus do not receive royalties, but they do reside on land that is recognized as impacted by the mine, and so receive benefits such as preferential employment. In short, a landowner is not a landowner is not a landowner, though most officially designated landowners are wealthier and more powerful than non-landowners.

PATRON-CLIENTISM AND TRAFFICKED WIVES

Some of Porgeran landowners' wealth is disseminated through the community, since there are strong cultural pressures to share (Biersack 2001, Jacka 2001). However, this sharing is often structured so as to form patron-client relations (Golub 2015: 147), so that landowners can gather around them less fortunate kith and kin who also serve as laborers and underlings and who owe their landowner patrons deference and allegiance. In return, landowners can bestow benefits such as money, use of land, attachment to artisanal and illegal mining operations, or even fictitious Ipili status for the purpose of gaining employment at the mine. Biersack, Jacka, and Golub all discuss the long-standing Ipili ethos of collecting people—related or not—on their land, and this practice has only intensified over the course of the mine's life. So, for example, Jacka found from census data in 1999 (that is, almost ten years after the mine opened) that 13 percent of the men living in the three Ipili hamlets that he surveyed were men who had married into the group, and fully 33 percent had no kinship relation whatsoever to the landowners—that is, altogether 46 percent of male residents were outsiders. In sum, as Golub puts it, "Each Ipili household has become something of a rentier operation in miniature, with its own line of immigrant clients" (2015: 148). With long-standing ties to Ipili groups, Huli make up a significant portion of these immigrant clients, and, because of sociopolitical turmoil and the collapse of public services in the Tari area (discussed in the next chapter), it is likely that this proportion increased over the 2000s (PEAK 2011).

Golub and Jacka both observe that landowners tend to be polygynous and that they marry strategically. For example, a landowner may marry a Porgeran woman from one of the twenty-three subclans to which he cannot claim membership in order to gain benefits through an in-law status, but he may also make a point of marrying women from remote rural areas, including in Huli territory, in order to acquire agricultural laborers. As Huli women who have lived in Porgera witheringly (but enviously) report, none of the female vegetable sellers in the Porgera main market belong to landowning families. "Women from landowner families don't do garden work," I was repeatedly told. "They don't even know how anymore. They just live off money." Thus, landowners seek out rural-born wives who will do this labor. Furthermore, Huli immigrant clients may seek to solidify their relationships with landowners by offering them their rural female kin as possible wives. Rural Huli families do not generally understand the great variability in landowner wealth: when they hear the term "landowner," the image they conjure up is of the extremely wealthy man who owns Land Cruisers and an electrified relocation house. This increases their willingness to marry off their daughters to Porgeran landowners they have never met.

It is these sociopolitical dynamics that produce HIV vulnerabilities not only for people living in Porgera, but also for people, especially women, from satellite population areas, such as Tari. Like Pamela, whose story started this chapter, two other women I interviewed were also essentially given in tribute by their kin to Porgeran landowners, and, like Pamela, they were from very remote areas, and their parents were offered bridewealth in amounts that were extremely high compared to the norm in these rural areas. Their parents therefore assented, with bridegroom sight unseen, despite arranged marriages being untraditional and normally frowned upon (marriages are sometimes arranged, but most parents would insist on getting to know the groom before agreeing, and usually the bride-to-be's opinion is sought). In each case, much as Pamela asserts, "it was a con" in the sense that the young women were told they would live lives of ease and that the marriage would take them away from onerous agricultural labor, but they found, to their dismay, that they were expected to spend their days much as they had in their natal homes: planting, weeding, and harvesting great swathes of sweet potato fields. Indeed, they realized quickly that they had been chosen precisely because they were from remote rural areas and it was consequently assumed that they were habituated to arduous physical work and were more likely to be obedient. They described their landowner husbands as autocratic, sometimes very generous, often unfaithful, and sometimes violent.

All three were told that their husband's goodwill to their resident kin depended on them remaining in the marriage (see also Jacka 2015: 126). Since these kin were essentially clients of the patron landowner, and dependent on him for economic opportunities and their very ability to stay in Porgera, they were unwilling to help these women leave their abusive marriages. Both Pamela and Kelapi, whose narrative is below, did eventually flee their situations, but on their own and without assistance from kin.

In Pamela's case, neighbors to whom she had always been generous observed her increasing sickliness, grew worried about her, and gave her enough money to get home by PMV. But as Pamela told it:

> After a month went by he sent bus fare and I came back. [Why did you go back?!] He threatened my kin. He said if I didn't come back he would kill Tari men living in Porgera. And I was afraid that he would hurt my relatives or that he would kill other men from Tari and that it would cause trouble (a common euphemism for tribal fighting). So I went back.
>
> But I was really sick—I had terrible diarrhea and ulcers inside my nose, and my nose swelled up. I was afraid I was dying, so I actually wanted to go back to Porgera so I could go to the hospital there, and they could find out what was wrong with me. (At that time Paiam Hospital in Porgera was reputed to have better services than most other hospitals in the region.) It was hard for me to travel. I had constant

diarrhea, so how was I going to sit on a PMV for hours and hours? But I made it back to Porgera, and after a few days my husband said, "Okay, let's go to the hospital and get a blood test."

But when we got there he said that only I would get a blood test. And it took me a long time to figure out, but he didn't ask for a blood test for himself because he'd already had one. In fact he'd known for a while, but never told me that he was HIV-positive. The nurses all knew him there—they knew he was positive. He tricked me. He knew all along that he had probably infected me and he was just pretending that he didn't know. I was furious, so, so furious. "This is your fault," I said. "This comes from you fucking lots of women." This was in 2011. I started taking ART in Porgera at Paiam Hospital. In 2012, I came back to Tari, and I have not been back to Porgera since.

Kelapi's story is similar to Pamela's:

I traveled with an uncle to Porgera, and then I married a man in Porgera. [How did you meet him?] He lived next door—we lived on his land. [So you had talked to him and knew him?] No. I just stayed at home and I fried lamb flaps to sell.[6] And one day he came to our house and he pulled me (a euphemism for rape) and forced me to go marry him. And I thought it would be ok—he looked like a good, healthy man. But I didn't know he already had a wife, and she was sick, and so he had sent her back to her village. . . . . .

[So you mean his wife was sick with AIDS?] Yes, she had contracted HIV, and she gave it to him, and then he sent her back to her village. [And this man, your husband, did he know that he had this sickness when he came and pulled you?] Yes, I think he knew, or at least he suspected. He conspired with my uncle's wife. They conspired that when I was home frying lamb flaps he would come rape me. . . . And he came to our house drunk. Everyone in Porgera was afraid of him because he was a landowner and also a well-known criminal. And he came charging in, and he sent the meat and the frying pan flying across the room. And then he took out K700 from his shoe, and he gave it to my uncle's wife. And then he took me to his house. And when I tried to come home, she lied to everyone and said, "I'm not going to have some woman living in my house who fools around and lets men into the house when no one is home. Go live with him—you can't live here." . . . .

And my uncle and his kin felt they couldn't do anything because he was a Porgera landowner, and he allowed them to live on his land. And he threatened to knife them and evict them, so they were afraid and did nothing. [I see. It wasn't their land and they were afraid?] Yes, and I was afraid he would hurt them, so I just went with him. And I thought that since he was a wealthy, powerful man my life would be okay. [I see. Did you try to run away?] Run away and do what? Go where? It wasn't my land—where would I go? How would I get back to Tari? I had no money. And I worried that if I ran away or tried to hide or ask my kin for money, he would come after them, threaten them, knife them. I was afraid for them, so I just stayed. I was afraid he would hurt my family. And I was also afraid that if he hurt them they would blame me. He was a bad man—a criminal. So I stayed put. . . . .

[How long did you live with him?] Two years and some months. I had a baby boy. He died when he was four months old. [Was it AIDS or something else?]

It was AIDS. Think about it—I married this man who had AIDS, and he must have infected me, and so the baby died. We took him to Paiam Hospital, but at that time people didn't talk about AIDS. There wasn't a Care Centre there yet, and the clinical staff didn't talk openly about AIDS. And there was no medicine. So even if you got a blood test they wouldn't tell you if you were positive or not. . . . But my baby was always sick—his mouth had lots of sores inside and he had diarrhea. He was big when he was born, but he lost weight fast, and then he died.

So I went back to the hospital on my own and got my blood tested. . . . When I came for the result, they handed me a piece of paper that said, "Reactive." And I had no idea what this meant. And so I asked, "Reactive? What does reactive mean?" But they wouldn't tell me or explain it. . . . So I went back home and I gave K20 to a man who worked at the hospital in a different department, and I gave him the paper and asked him what "reactive" meant. He was afraid, and he said, "I'm afraid. I'm not supposed to say. I work in a different department, and if they found out that I told you they would take me to court." All he would say was, "You need to eat well. You should eat lots of fruit, eat nutritious food." But I had heard that they always tell people with AIDS to eat lots of fruit, and so I was sure that I had AIDS.[7] And so I ran away from my husband and came home to Tari. . . . . [And was your husband showing any symptoms?] I don't know. People have told me he is now on ART, but I don't know. I did ask him, but all he would say is, "I'm a company man—I don't have AIDS." He was a landowner and, you know, the landowners are given jobs easily and don't really have to do anything. And I asked him, but he got angry, and all he would say is, "I'm the kind of man who works for the company. I'm a company man! I'm a landowner! I don't have AIDS!"

Here again we see that the patron-client relationships between Porgeran landowners and Huli immigrants are solidified through marriage so that the woman given (or, in this case, forcibly taken) as tribute becomes a kind of lynchpin: her flight could result in the expulsion of her kin or, if the threats of these landowner husbands are to be believed, in retaliatory violence against them. Also significant in this story is the apparent complicity of Kelapi's uncle's wife, who was paid for her help in arranging the sexual assault and forced marriage, and then made it impossible for Kelapi to return to her uncle's home by ruining her reputation (i.e., telling others that she was "the kind of woman who lets men into the house when no one else is home"). This kind of collusion in sexual violence, done with the aim of forcing a young woman to act as the link to an influential patron, is rare to my knowledge; however, I have come across other cases, which similarly entailed not only cooperation, but orchestration, by an older woman who was trusted by the victim (Wardlow 2006b). While female solidarity is valued by Huli women, it is also easily fragmented by other interests and allegiances, and often takes a back seat to generational authority.

Also significant in Kelapi's narrative is her husband's consternation at his own (unadmitted) HIV-positive status. The few HIV-positive men I interviewed—indeed, especially the successful ones who had salaried jobs—often seemed shocked at their positive diagnoses, despite histories of unprotected sex with many partners, and they exhibited this same sort of angry incredulous bluster. ("I'm a company man! I'm a landowner! I don't have AIDS!") In the case of Kelapi's husband, his assertion may simply have been an attempt to maintain masculine dignity in the face of female accusation. But, I suspect that the element of disbelief is genuine, at least for some men. As many ethnographers of highlands Papua New Guinea have observed, a man's socio-moral identity is often said to be exhibited "on the skin," positing a direct relationship between one's inner capacities and qualities and one's external appearance (A. Strathern 1975, M. Strathern 1979, O'Hanlon 1989). In particular, social power and charisma are thought to express themselves through a powerful and vigorous body. For a man who has achieved the epitome of success—being a wealthy landowner, accumulating immigrant clients, having a salaried job with "the company"—being diagnosed with an illness associated with emaciation, loss of bodily continence, and social ostracism—might, in fact, have seemed impossible.

CONCLUSION

Most important in Pamela's and Kelapi's stories, and perhaps insufficiently empha-sized in the existing literature about Papua New Guinea landowners, is the way that the relations between landowner patrons and immigrant clients can rest on a foundation of gender inequality, gendered moral duty, and gendered violence. Not all immigrants provide wives to their patron landowners, of course, but marriage is, for both Huli and Ipili, the best way to produce enduring relations into the next generation. Marriage ideally creates children who are "in between" the two fami-lies (Biersack 1995), thus linking them together and creating obligations between them. All of this depends, of course, on women agreeing to such marriages and staying in them, which, as we've seen, can be secured through violence and threats of violence. Both Pamela and Kelapi when considering escape weighed not only the possible violent consequences to themselves, but also the violence that their husbands might inflict on their kin, and how their kin might inflict violence on them for undermining the patron-client bond.

Indeed, in both Kelapi's and Pamela's cases, it was only the exceptionalism of AIDS as a dreaded disease that induced them to run away. A husband's violence or extramarital escapades weren't sufficient reason, but being infected with HIV by him was. At the time when Kelapi and Pamela were diagnosed, knowledge about the new availability of antiretrovirals was not widespread; thus, both women initially believed their husbands had given them a "death sentence," as Pamela said. Thinking they would soon die, both women finally felt justified in returning home to their natal kin. Moreover, both women were furious about the deaths of their infants and the squandering of their reproductive labor. As Pamela bit-terly retorted when I asked if her husband had demanded his bridewealth back after her escape, "Why would we return bridewealth? I gave him a child, but he threw it away on AIDS," by which she meant that she had done her reproductive duty as a wife (that is, fulfilled the obligations of the bridewealth payment), and it was ultimately her husband's reckless sexual behavior that had killed their child. Anticipating that future marital sex would only result in the same heartbreaking, dismal end intensified both women's determination to leave.[8]

This chapter also demonstrates that resource-extraction sites—or "rural development enclaves"—produce gendered HIV vulnerability in multiple ways. Of the eight HIV-positive women I interviewed whose infections were linked to resource-extraction sites, three were infected by landowner husbands, three by husbands who worked at Moro, and one most likely by her husband who worked as a policeman in Porgera. The eighth was the half-sister of a Porgeran landowner, whose husband courted her in order to gain access to her half-brother, who eventually got him a job as a security guard in Porgera, a case that demonstrates that landowners not only seek out wives from would-be clients, but also use their female kin to cultivate clients.

Finally, it is important to note that Papua New Guinea's policies guiding resource extraction—for example, the FIFO model of using labor and the identification of landowner groups for mining benefits—shape the sexual economy in Porgera in ways that make the profile of HIV vulnerability there overlap with, but also differ from, the existing anthropological model of HIV risk at mine sites, which is based on data from the migrant labor–dependent, deep elevator-shaft mining of South Africa. The South African mining model has become somewhat canonical in medical anthropology, not only because of the innovative and compelling nature of Campbell's and others' work, but also because this work continues a long lineage of scholarly research on mining, migration, and disease in South Africa (e.g., Packard 1989, Marks 2006, Basu et al. 2009). Papua New Guinea's mining geology, history, and policy environment has its own particularities, which create a somewhat different sexual economy and thus different gendered vulnerabilities to HIV.

Also important to Porgera's HIV risk milieu is its pervasive violence between numerous and wide-ranging stakeholders (company security staff, landowners, non-landowners, etc.). Violence in Porgera is often represented as "traditional" by mining managers, and this ideological representation of violence around the mine as "tribal" and "customary" further entrenches the sometimes explicit construction of the mining company as civilized and the local populace as savage, which serves both to absolve the company of responsibility and to legitimate redoubling the protection of the mining enclave. Much as James Ferguson suggested in "Seeing Like An Oil Company" (2005), increased violence among Porgeran people has justified increased militarization of the mining area.

Women are often victims of this violent environment. International attention has focused on PJV security guards' rape of Porgeran women (Human Rights Watch 2011); however, it has mostly escaped notice that women like Pamela and Kelapi are essentially victims of trafficking, duped or forced into marrying

Porgeran landowner husbands. It would be incorrect, I think, to see the incidents of rape by PJV security guards as discrete or anomalous phenomena to be bracketed off analytically from other kinds of gender violence that occur in the mining environment, such as forced or coerced marriages to landowner patrons. Rather, sexual violence on the part of security personnel and the tribute of women to landowners both stem from social stratification instantiated or intensified by the mine: male security guards, tasked with securing the extractive enclave, come to view local inhabitants as unruly threats who need to be disciplined and punished, including through sexual violence. And landowners, consolidating their position in the local hierarchy, come to see dependent migrants as subordinates who need to know their place, including through coerced and forced sex and marriage.

This is a male hierarchy consisting of male mine managers, male landowners, male mine workers, male security guards, and male migrant dependents. Women often serve as pawns in this masculine social field: they enable men to forge alliances with others, they are offered as tokens of male tribute, and sexual violence against them is a potent cautionary reminder to their kin of their vulnerability to men higher up in the hierarchy. That HIV prevalence is higher in such a social field is not surprising.

2

State Abandonment, Sexual Violence, and Transactional Sex

Sarah was infected with HIV when the PMV she was taking from Mendi back to Tari was held up at gunpoint by a group of Nipa men, and the female passengers were raped. This was a painful, stumbling interview because she was sullen and glum, and my desire to interview her clashed with my urge to console her. One of the youngest of the women I interviewed, she was also one of the most despondent, asserting that she couldn't imagine marrying or having children, because she couldn't imagine having sex or anyone wanting to marry her. She described her own HIV-positive body as abject, and she was revolted by the idea that she might marry a man who was also living with HIV.

She had been sent by her mother to buy betel nut and wholesale cigarettes to sell back in Tari. People often preferred to buy goods in Mendi or Mt. Hagen because they were cheaper there than in Tari; even taking the cost of a PMV round trip into account, a bit more profit could be made. Her mother didn't go herself because she suffered from chronic back and leg pain and didn't feel she could undergo the jarring trip on a hard wooden bench over a rutted dirt road. The region being thick with interethnic ties of marriage and friendship, within days word got back to Sarah's family that her rapist was rumored to be HIV-positive. By that time, MSF had a well-established project providing clinical care and counselling for survivors of sexual violence, and Sarah didn't live far from Tari hospital; however, she hadn't sought care from them and said that she had never heard of them.[1] Two years after the incident, Sarah was still angry that her kin had not demanded compensation or retaliated for the attack. "One of my brothers—a drug-body (i.e., a marijuana smoker)—raped a Nipa woman who came here to sell betel nut. He said it was for retaliation. I don't know. Then they got married. That's all that happened," she muttered. In fact, the PMV holdup itself had been retaliation for the murder of a Nipa man in Port Moresby, so it is possible that Huli leaders didn't want to escalate the conflict any further. For Sarah, the decision not to seek revenge rankled.

Sarah's might seem like a clear-cut case in terms of where to allocate blame for her infection—the Nipa men who held up her PMV and raped her and other female passengers—but, in fact, Sarah asserted that her mother was the primary *tene* (root or cause). Unpredictable outbreaks of hostilities with the Nipa were the way of the world, she suggested, but her mother should have known—did, in fact, know—that Sarah was too young to be sent on a daylong journey on a route that was plagued by crime: "I told her, 'It is your fault that I have this sickness. You were the one who did this. You were the one who told me I had to go to Mendi and buy those goods. It is because of you that I was on the road going back and forth and I found this sickness. What are you going to do about it?'" (Here Sarah was implying that her mother should give her compensation.) Furious, she had briefly left her mother's household and moved in with her father's kin, who were threatening to take her mother to village court and demand compensation. The charge would have been something like reckless endangerment that not only put Sarah in harm's way, but also diminished her value, since few men would knowingly marry an HIV-positive woman, and her father's kin might thus never receive bridewealth for her. In the end, her father decided that he would only pursue a compensation case against Sarah's mother if Sarah died, and since she was thriving physically on ARVs, this didn't seem likely.[2]

. . .

The armed robbery of Sarah's PMV occurred in 2011, a period in which such incidents were diminishing, largely because of the increased police presence on the road between Tari and Mendi intended to protect drivers and cargo destined for the LNG (such protections had not been there in the past). The late 1990s and early 2000s were a far more dangerous and tumultuous period, and in this chapter I examine that earlier era, a time of sociopolitical conflict, pervasive crime, and governmental abandonment that produced HIV vulnerability through increases in both sexual violence and sex work, as well as much reduced health services.

A FAILED ELECTION AND ITS AFTERMATH

Until 2012, when it was officially cut in two, with the western half becoming Hela Province, Southern Highlands Province was Papua New Guinea's most populous, and one of the largest by territory. There had long been tensions between east and west, at least since 1980, when the Huli provincial premier, Andrew Andaija, died in a plane crash, and many Huli alleged that ethnic groups in the east had used sorcery to bring down the plane. Many people trace the tensions further back, however, insisting that Michael Somare, the prime minister at the time of Independence in 1975 (and again from 2002 to 2011), had broken his promise to the Huli that they would receive their own province, instead creating a province that did not accord with their own understanding of the proper boundaries and its cosmologically ordained ethnic composition. The position of provincial premier (and later governor) of Southern Highlands Province had therefore long been hotly contested between the Huli and the Mendi, the other large ethnic group in the province, with everyone assuming that a Mendi governor would bring development to the Mendi and allow the Huli to languish, while a Huli governor would do the opposite. Long-simmering tensions boiled over in 1997 after Dick Mune, a former governor belonging to the Nipa, a Mendi sub-group, died in a car accident. This time, Nipa people blamed Anderson Agiru, the Huli governor who had succeeded Mune, alleging sorcery. The only road between Tari and Mendi, the provincial capital of Southern Highlands Province, goes through Nipa territory, and Nipa people were determined not only to rob Huli vehicles, but to prevent any and all goods and supplies from reaching Tari.

The situation only grew worse during and after the next national election in 2002. Agiru had been suspended as governor in 2000 on grounds of corruption and mismanagement of funds, and was not permitted to run, a ruling that many Huli found humiliating and described as national discrimination against them as a people. Haley and May note that in the lead-up to the election, candidates in Southern Highlands Province stockpiled weapons and distributed them to their supporters, and that one "prominent candidate flew in cartons of semi-automatic weapons purchased in China while on an official government visit, so that his supporters might usurp control of the elections on polling day" (Haley and May 2007: 12; see also Alpers 2004). There was widespread election malfeasance throughout the country, and, in Southern Highlands Province, ballot boxes were stuffed or stolen, a candidate was kidnapped and held for ransom, people were intimidated or forced into voting for specific candidates, and a few people were killed. The conflict was not only between the east and west of the province, but also between candidates vying for positions within electorates. The elections were deemed to have failed in six of Southern Highlands Province's nine electorates, and no governor was elected, essentially leaving the province without a government until new elections could be held (Dorpar and Macpherson 2007). When supplementary elections were held ten months later, with two thousand additional police and soldiers sent in to maintain order, the process was still compromised by fraud and violence, even though a new governor, Hami Yawari, who was neither Huli nor Mendi, was elected.

The consequences of these ongoing conflicts, the failed 2002 elections, and the lack of a provincial government were profound and enduring. Nipa groups continued to hold up Huli PMVs at gunpoint, sometimes assaulting and raping passengers. PMVs and government vehicles carrying supplies for schools or health centers were often robbed, and throughout my six months in Tari in 2004, the hospital was usually without essential medicines and supplies. Stores had difficulty maintaining their stocks, and prices went up, because the only way to ensure safety on the road was to pay for a police escort, a cost that was passed on to consumers. Ongoing roadblocks and robberies also meant that fuel often didn't reach Tari, and as a result, government employees, including the police, were sometimes unable to carry out their duties in the district.

Guns continued to flood into the area. Days before I flew to Tari in February 2004, EMTV, the national TV network, reported that the Port Moresby airport's luggage security scanner, which had been broken for weeks but was finally fixed, had caught two men trying to bring guns, ammunition, and bullet-proof vests to Tari. How many guns had been flown in before the scanner was repaired no one knew, and police checkpoints into the province were not much of a deterrent. With the deterioration of services, the lack of economic opportunities, bitterness about the election results, and the influx of guns, crime within Huli territory increased. It quickly became conventional wisdom that rural households had to have someone at home at all times or risk being robbed. I once met an elderly woman who had been designated to stay at home when everyone else was away, but fell ill and had to stay overnight at the hospital. When she returned home, "everything was gone, even the scrap of towel for cleaning the baby's bottom."

Crime in town also became flagrant. In 2002, for example, a gang looted Bromley's, the one large store in Tari, for three days straight. As described to me, the men kept armed watch while their female kin hauled out everything of high value, such as electronic goods. Outnumbered and outgunned, the police were routed after a brief shootout. Then there was a free-for-all until the store was empty. My friends recalled it as three days of terror and delight: everyone was afraid of what the gang might do next, but, in the end, they had distributed cans of meat, cartons of instant noodle soups, and boxes of biscuits to everyone. Many people felt that since they couldn't afford most of the goods in the store anyway, they didn't care if it was robbed; it was "the missionaries' store," they said, meaning it stocked goods that expatriate missionaries bought and that only they could afford (imported pastas, breakfast cereal, cheese). This store never reopened, and the one bank in town and the post office also closed because of armed robberies.

With no banking services in Tari, and the persistent threat of holdups on the road to Mendi, public servants were unable to access their pay. Soon teachers and health workers began to leave, which led to the closure of schools and health centers, which led to yet more departures. Public servants didn't want to stay in a place where they didn't feel safe, where their children were unable to go to school, and where they couldn't access their pay. In 2004, the hospital, which was supposed to have 97 employees, only had 15, and no doctor (which meant it didn't actually qualify as a hospital). The employees who remained often didn't show up for work; without the most basic medicines and supplies, there was not much they could do, and morale was poor.

Tribal fighting also increased during this period. Crime and tribal fighting are complexly tied together, and when one increases, the other tends to also; indeed, it can be difficult to distinguish between the two. One might assume that the armed holdup of a PMV should be categorized as crime, since passengers are robbed and assaulted, but the intent to harm may be part of an ongoing political conflict, as between the Huli and Nipa (cf. Roscoe 2014). Conversely, crimes such as murder or rape may ultimately result in a larger violent conflict between clans associated with victim and perpetrator. For example, after the village court case regarding Tabitha's sexual assault (discussed below), a man from the alleged rapist's clan publicly maligned Tabitha and, with tempers high because the dispute was not yet resolved, men from Tabitha's side attacked him with machetes, nearly severing his arms. This precipitated tribal conflict, with the two sides burning down one another's houses.

Furthermore, ongoing tribal fighting may result in crimes, such as robbery, in order to raise money, either for guns to escalate the conflict, or for the homicide compensation payments to end it. Rather than a concerted attack, group conflicts sometimes take the form of a series of individual criminal assaults—for example, the murder or rape of someone from the enemy group—and retaliation for a crime may take place during tribal fighting. A public servant told me that he had saved for years to build his own house, but that the very expensive recently installed windows and solar panels had been stolen; knowing the young men who were responsible and aware that their clan was embroiled in warfare, he had paid young men from the other side to target them, their families, and their homes. "'But bring back the solar panels,' I told them," he said.

The small police force in Tari was unable to deter this vicious cycle of crime and warfare, and the district administrator was reluctant to request a police mobile squad detachment without a concomitant rebuilding of public services. He knew that some of the crime was motivated by anger at the profound deterioration of health and education services, as well as the failure to maintain roads or create economic opportunities, and he believed that the potentially brutal use of police to intimidate and jail people might only further antagonize the populace. He wanted to try to restore services before bringing in additional police reinforcements, but was engaged in regular discussions with Porgera Joint Venture management, some of whom disagreed with this strategy and wanted to send in more police immediately.

Porgera Joint Venture was in a position to exert some influence over this debate because the Porgera mine in Enga Province is powered by a natural gas plant located in Hides, seventy-eight kilometers south of the mine, squarely in Hela Province. Two hundred and twenty-eight enormous electrical pylons—known as the Hides transmission line—snake their way from Hides to Porgera. The mine is thus dependent on a source of power that is located in a different province among Huli who not only do not benefit from the mine (i.e., receive no royalties or preferential employment), but also do not receive electricity from the transmission line. Without this electricity, the mine cannot operate, and in 2002, Huli men sabotaged thirty-eight of the pylons, closing the mine for three months.

Toppling Hides transmission line pylons in order to express complaint is, in fact, a long-standing tactic on the part of Huli groups: when I first arrived at my field site for my doctoral research in 1995, I beheld the charred remains of still smoldering houses, burned by local police. Reportedly acting on instructions from PJV, they had resorted to violent measures, including beatings and house burnings, in order to coerce local leaders into turning over the young men who had recently felled two of the pylons. In 2004, Huli friends and PJV staff told me that the 2002 pylon sabotage was intended less as an expression of resentment of PJV and more as a message to the government that the lack of services had become intolerable. With their elected representatives unwilling to visit Tari to hear their grievances, they had shrewdly decided to target an important source of revenue for the state, its second-largest gold mine. They correctly surmised that this sabotage would quickly and effectively get the attention of both government and corporation. As Alice Street has pointed out, governmental neglect can motivate people's increasingly desperate attempts to "force the state to recognize its obligations towards them" (Street 2012: 3). During this period, roughly from 1999 to 2004, the state was experienced by Huli less as a monolith deploying technologies of legibility and discipline (Scott 1988), and more as an absent entity that people had to compel to see them, to recognize their miseries and needs.

PJV responded this time, not with intimidation and violence, but by assuming some of the duties associated with an effective state. For example, it established a small Community Relations Office in Tari, staffed by a network of male community liaison officers from the various landowning groups along the Hides transmission line, and it used Papua New Guinea's tax credit scheme to maintain goodwill in the area by building schools and maintaining roads and bridges.[3] With discretionary funds available to them for community projects they deemed worthwhile, expatriate PJV managers in Tari gave money and other assistance to sports teams, women's groups, and youth groups ("youth groups" in this context consisted mostly of young men who had formed a group for the sole purpose of being hired for PJV projects, such as cleaning Tari town of litter or cutting the grass on the air strip). And families who owned land on which an electrical pylon had been erected were given a "security" payment—a new payment every six months of K650 per tower provided it had not been vandalized. PJV also sometimes attempted to "turn" known saboteurs, deliberately recruiting some of them to be community liaison officers. The main goal of all of this, of course, was to keep the towers up so that gold could continue to be excavated. In 2004, the PJV community relations office was the only source of economic opportunity in Tari. Every weekday there was a twenty-five-yard or longer line of petitioners outside the ten-foot-tall gate hoping to gain an audience with a PJV staff member who might help with transport to a functioning hospital, funds for school fees, letters of introduction or recommendation, or supplies to begin a chicken project or some other income-generating endeavor.

STATE ABANDONMENT: "TARI IS A NO-GO ZONE"

Seeking to "unsettle conceptualizations of the state as a singular, rational, and stable entity" (Pinker and Harvey 2018: 17), anthropologists have examined the state's ontological nature with renewed vigor, often citing a seminal paper by Phillip Abrams (1988) questioning the reality of the state and arguing that it is best understood as an ideological project. Christopher Krupa and David Nugent observe that "one of the most enduring conventions of state realism is a centrifocal imaginary. That is, state power is regarded as something that is concentrated in various bureaucratic-administrative centers, from which it radiates outward across national-territorial space" (Krupa and Nugent 2015: 10). Eschewing the narrative of "state realism" and attempting to disrupt this centrifocal imaginary, they argue that an ethnographic approach to the state should investigate how "the state as phenomenological reality is produced . . . in local encounters at the everyday level" (Aretxaga 2003: 393) and "conjured into being in the context of the minutiae of everyday life" (Krupa and Nugent 2015: 9). In other words, what specifically do people experience in their daily lives that enables them to imagine and construct the state in particular ways?

Some scholars who have adopted this phenomenological ethnographic approach have observed that state power typically extends beyond the places and agencies in which it is officially located, making the state "unsiteable" (Navaro-Yashin 2002: 3). In other words, while the state may be imagined as embodied in particular offices or institutions, its practices and representatives can in fact exert power outside and beyond these. Moreover, the state often exists most powerfully through its "affective life"—that is, through "the ways desire, hope, and fear may simultaneously invest us in projects of state" (Krupa and Nugent 2015: 14). The state thus comes to exist for and in people, not only through internalized state discourses, but also through people's aspirations and utopian hopes. Moreover, "attending to affect . . . provides insights into how the state interchangeably materializes and disappears—contingently yet consequentially—in everyday interactions," Mateusz Laszczkowski and Madeleine Reeves argue (2018: 10). In other words, the state can be experienced as an unreliable affective interlocutor, sometimes present and attentive, sometimes distant and oblivious. Investigating the land claims of South Africans dispossessed of property during the apartheid era, and the onerous forms that claimants were required to fill out, Christiaan Beyers calls this dynamic an "affective deficit" and suggests that the state creates cathexis in people by building up their affective desires, but can then unexpectedly seem to vanish from the relationship; there is "a large discrepancy between the desire manifested in narratives inscribed on claim forms and what the claims process yields . . . the sense of anticipation in filling out forms is met with flat nothingness over time. The dialogic flow of affectivity in language meets a dead end," and although the state's affective deficit—and its failures to provide effective restitution—can lead to cynicism, in many cases, it "is itself productive in a sense, since the desire for recognition is sustained by its deferment" (Beyers 2018: 77–78). In other words, the state creates itself as an entity by producing longing, unfulfilled desires, and intimations of future improvement.

In Tari, during this tumultuous period, the Papua New Guinea state was affectively present (in people's fear and anger) largely through its disappearance—that is, through the sites and institutions in which people expected it to be, but it no longer was. It was "unsiteable," not because it exceeded the sites it was expected to occupy, but because it had evacuated them. One afternoon in 2004, for example, I carried out participant observation at the hospital in an empty outpatient area, an area that five years before and five years later, was easily packed all day long with hundreds of patients. I sat for hours with a handful of patients, and nobody came. I then wandered through the empty old maternity ward, spattered with bloodstains and littered with rusted equipment, and then through the empty "new" maternity ward, which had sat unused for years, because it was never connected to the water supply, its pink curtains gathering dust and dead insects. Similarly, only a few police were posted to Tari in early 2004, and a question that queasily made its way through town every day was whether any of them were in the station. No police meant that there might be more robberies at the main market or holdups of PMVs.

"For the majority of Papua New Guineans . . . the state exists primarily as an absence. . . . The decrepit condition or lack of state infrastructure such as roads, schools or health centres suggests to those living in rural areas that they have been forgotten or betrayed by politicians," Alice Street notes (2012: 16). One might thus characterize much of rural Papua New Guinea as experiencing a perpetual "affective deficit" (as well as a services and infrastructure deficit) in relation to the state. In Tari, however, the state was experienced, not simply as an affective deficit or absence, but as a terrifying and punishing abandonment. Not only did government workers abscond, but the state's physical infrastructure also began to disappear. The mattresses at the hospital were stolen, for example. And at night I was often woken by the sound of men prying sheets of metal roofing off of the abandoned courthouse nearby; little by little, the metal roofing disappeared, then windowpanes, then wooden beams. Segments of the Tari airport fence went missing, and people began using the runway area for grazing animals during the day and drinking parties at night. With sheep and beer bottles littering the airstrip, Air Niugini ceased its flights.

The situation was not merely a case of Tari being geographically or discursively located in the "margins of the state," conceptualized inter alia as "the peripheries seen to form natural containers for people considered insufficiently socialized into the law" (Das and Poole 2004: 9). There is no doubt that the Huli have been, and continue to be, seen by government elites as not just insufficiently socialized into the law, but as arrogantly rejecting it. Nevertheless, the concept of marginality, with its suggestion of languishing neglect or irrelevancy, does not quite capture the active abandonment that was taking place at this time. On a visit to Port Moresby, I was told by staff at the National AIDS Council (NAC) that Tari had been unofficially declared "a no-go zone": fearful of being abducted and held for ransom, politicians refused to visit it, and NGOs refused to send their employees there.[4] In hushed tones, staff at the NAC and at some NGOs said that the province was being "punished": if the people couldn't learn to participate in an orderly democratic process, they wouldn't get any governance at all. And one PJV manager informed me that he'd heard politicians in Port Moresby say they wished they could build a wall around the province and forget about it.

One consequence of this was that the HIV prevention programming that was taking place in other provinces was not implemented in the Tari area. I would make the occasional trip to Port Moresby and learn from NAC staff about innovative youth group or peer education projects happening elsewhere, but no basic HIV awareness, let alone more creative or targeted interventions, was planned for Tari. Similarly, condoms were almost completely unavailable. Some enterprising men occasionally went to Mendi or Mt. Hagen, stocked up on condoms there, and sold them to other men back in Tari for a profit, but they were not available at Tari stores. Health facilities that had them only provided them to married men who said they needed them for family planning purposes, guided by the theory that refusing to distribute them for other reasons would discourage pre- and extramarital sex. I therefore brought large cartons of condoms back from the National AIDS Council and gave them to my four male field assistants and male PJV staff to sell or distribute as they saw fit.

In April 2004, the Papua New Guinea state reappeared in force. Forty mobile squad police were sent to Tari in response to two events. First, the district administrator's truck was burned, which was interpreted as a direct assault on the government. Second, the gang responsible for much of the more flagrant crime in Tari abducted two PJV employees (they let them go after using them to gain entry to PJV facilities so that they could refuel).[5] The police chased after them, and their leader, David Agini, and most of the members died, either shot by the police or killed when they crashed their truck. Government officials feared that Agini's kin and supporters might retaliate by attacking the police or burning down government buildings, and so a mobile squad was sent. As noted in chapter 1, given their reputation for thuggish behavior, mobile squads are often feared. In this case, however, they were respectful, and their presence successfully brought peace to the area for the duration of their stay. When they left a few months later, hundreds of people lined the roads through and out of town, and wept as their trucks drove past. The state was given palpable affective life with tears shed as it disappeared yet again.

The governmental abandonment of this period, from the end of the 1990s until the mid 2000s, exacerbated HIV vulnerabilities in Tari, not only through the state's failure to carry out HIV awareness and prevention activities, but also by creating a social environment in which violent, coercive, and transactional sex inevitably flourished. I divide the following discussion into two rough categories, sexual violence and transactional sex. In some cases these two categories are clear-cut: the rape at gunpoint of Sarah and other female PMV passengers involved no "transactional" give-and-take, only violent seizure. But some instances are less easily classified: one woman I interviewed in 2004 spoke of risking the road to Mendi because

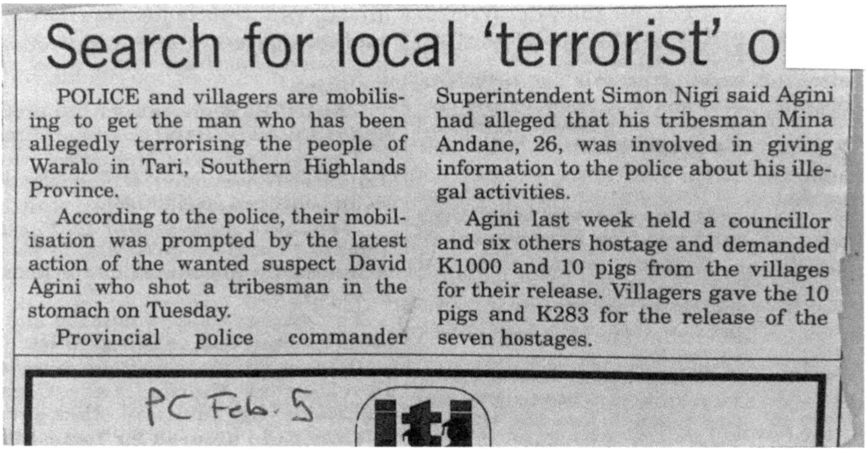

Search for local 'terrorist' o

POLICE and villagers are mobilising to get the man who has been allegedly terrorising the people of Waralo in Tari, Southern Highlands Province.

According to the police, their mobilisation was prompted by the latest action of the wanted suspect David Agini who shot a tribesman in the stomach on Tuesday.

Provincial police commander Superintendent Simon Nigi said Agini had alleged that his tribesman Mina Andane, 26, was involved in giving information to the police about his illegal activities.

Agini last week held a councillor and six others hostage and demanded K1000 and 10 pigs from the villages for their release. Villagers gave the 10 pigs and K283 for the release of the seven hostages.

PC Feb. 5

FIGURE 5. Clipping from the *Post Courier* newspaper about David Agini, February 5, 2004. Photo by author.

she desperately needed to call her brother, and there were no working phones in Tari (mobile phones did not arrive in Tari until 2008); once there, she agreed to sex with a public servant in exchange for the use of his phone. This episode raises the question: when men have the power to act as gatekeepers to needed goods and services, and demand sex in exchange for access to them, is this a transaction or violence? In short, even as I use the categories of sexual violence and transactional sex to analyze the sexual entanglements fostered by state abandonment, it is important to bear in mind that Tari itself, governmentally forsaken, had become a more brutal place, one that made these distinctions problematic (cf. Burnet 2012).

SEXUAL VIOLENCE

The Prevalence of Rape and Its Causes

It is difficult to know the prevalence of sexual violence in Tari, because unless a woman is badly injured, cases of sexual violence are generally not reported to the hospital or the police. This is in part because rape is conceptualized primarily as an appropriative violation against a family, necessitating revenge or compensation, and not as a traumatizing violation of the individual that may require clinical or psychological care. Going to the hospital is therefore usually considered unnecessary, and reporting to the police is often avoided, because they might interfere with a family's intentions to exact revenge.[6] Consequently, it is impossible to provide definitive numbers for sexual violence in the Tari area, its fluctuations over time, and how these fluctuations might correlate with political or socioeconomic changes.

That said, there is more information about this than one might expect, and it indicates very high levels of sexual violence in the Hela region during the early and mid 2000s. For one thing, a survey that investigated households' experiences of various violent crimes (domestic violence, armed robbery, sexual violence, etc.) found that in Southern Highlands Province in 2005, 8 percent of households said that a member had experienced sexual assault during the previous six months. Of these cases, 89 percent were in the province's Hela region (Haley and Muggah 2006: 46). Furthermore, my examination of injury-related medical records at Tari Hospital in April 2004 also showed very high levels of sexual violence at that time, with seven incidents of rape involving multiple attackers during just the first three months of that year. I made a point of examining the hospital injury records because I had been shocked to learn of four village court cases about rape taking place just within the immediate vicinity of my guesthouse, and I wanted to ascertain whether data were available that supported what people overwhelmingly described as a frightening increase in sexual violence. The cases most often seen by the hospital staff were those described as gang or pack rapes, often because the female victims were more badly injured during such incidents.

I copied the following notes from the records:

1. F, 17, pack rape by 3 men. Traveling with mother and sister.
2. F, 16, resisted. Multiple pocket knife wounds to back and head.
3. F, 20, pack rape by 4 men.
4. F, 17, pack rape by 3 men.
5. F, 23, 7 men pack rape. Also axe wound to head and bashed by guns when she tried to resist.
6. F, 65, pack rape by 6 men, midnight.
7. F, 21, pack rape by 5 men, 9 am.

The reasons for this increase in sexual violence were multiple. First and foremost was the increase in political conflict and the concomitant increase in crime, including rape. A number of scholars have analyzed the pervasiveness of sexual violence in conflict zones, demonstrating that rather than being seen as a symptom of anarchy or the breakdown of moral order, sexual violence should be understood as a deliberate strategy for terrorizing and humiliating the enemy (Seifert 1994, Enloe 2000, Turshen 2001, Meger 2010, Burnet 2012). These analyses have some relevance for understanding the situation in the Tari area during this period: women belonging to enemy groups are typically not killed, but they may be targeted for rape, with the intent of humiliating the enemy, instilling fear, and hemming in an enemy group in order to limit their economic activity. Fearful of attack, women will either flee an area or not stray outside family territory; either way, unable to access agricultural fields or markets, their economic contributions to family and clan are usually severely curtailed. In this sense, rape is used as a weapon of war in the Tari area.

That said, much of the literature analyzing sexual violence in conflict zones is not very apt to the situation in the Hela region during this period. Women were not abducted by enemy groups or forcibly impregnated by them, for example. And fighting did not necessarily or even often take place on a field of battle, but instead consisted of isolated and opportunistic acts: a male member of an enemy group might be killed while walking home alone after a night of drinking and gambling; a female member of an enemy group might be raped as she walked home from her garden at dusk. Individuals were sometimes chosen as targets because they represented powerful assets of the enemy—a trade-store owner or a highly educated man, for example. But they were also often chosen because they were vulnerable and easy targets; thus, women living alone might be chosen for home invasion and rape.

In the absence of an effective police force that could work to prevent and punish sexual violence and other crimes, people increasingly relied on their own family resources, especially their young men. For example, I repeatedly observed older women use threats of sexual violence against other women in order to deter property crime. Suspecting a family of robbing her fields or stealing her chickens, a senior woman might loudly ask when she encountered women from the family, "Do you think we don't have young men in our household? Do you think we won't send them? Do you think we can't take your pigs? Or your girls? Our young men are standing by." As noted in chapter 1, although female solidarity is valued by Huli women, it is often fragmented along lines of generation or kinship affiliation. Thus, older women seemed to have no qualms about threatening younger women belonging to enemy families with retaliation by their own young male kin.

Often the young men would, in fact, be standing silently in the background as these threats of retaliatory theft and rape were made. And they knew that such threats were not merely tactics of intimidation. Men were expected to follow through when their family members were assaulted, and violent retaliation was understood, not only as punishment for others' behavior, but also as a gift of revenge or protection to one's own kin. When there were rumors that a gang had threatened to rob me, more than one young male friend of mine tried to reassure me by promising that he would rape the sister of any man who attacked me. Though taken aback, I came to understand these promises for what they were: what little a young man could offer, and was expected to do, for women he wanted to defend (which is not to say that sexual assaults didn't also have other meanings in terms of male solidarity, masculine potency, and the re-inscription of sexual difference and male domination through sexual violence). And, in order to protect their families and property, older women were complicit in making and mobilizing these threats.

In short, during this chaotic period, sexual violence became a resource for punishing enemy incursions, and occasionally people even articulated a kind of calculus: in the repertoire of possible tactics for preventing or punishing encroachments by enemy groups or pilfering by bold neighbors, sexual violence

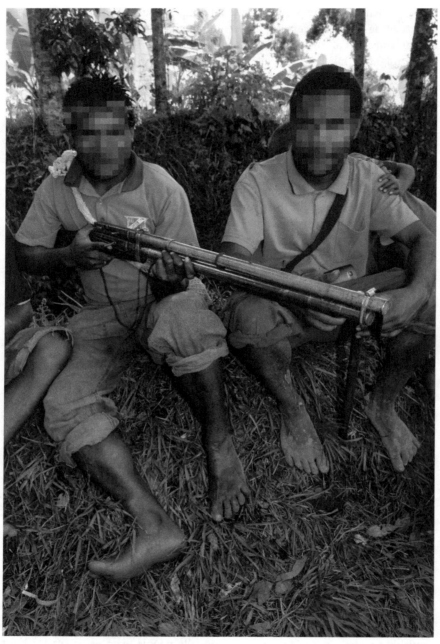

FIGURE 6. Two boys with a gun, faces pixelated for their protection. Photo by Kenneth I. MacDonald.

was worse than stealing pigs, but not nearly as bad as murder or armed assault. People deplored the increase in sexual violence and complained about young men "causing trouble," but they also wanted to be able to deploy these troublesome young men when necessary. Young men were thus not always acting autonomously when they started "trouble," and they were encouraged to maintain a state of masculine affective volatility, anger, and readiness for violence, including sexual violence.

Incidents of rape were sometimes highly polysemous in intent, however. Departing dramatically from the existing literature about sexual violence in conflict zones, where it has been argued that women from enemy groups are objects of hatred and that rape serves to further dehumanize them (Meger 2010, Seifert 1994), it was sometimes the case that a young man wanting to avenge the rape of female kin might choose to assault a young woman for whom he had romantic feelings, hoping both to meet others' expectations of revenge, but also to bring about a marriage for himself, since marriage is one way of resolving sexual assault disputes. For example, when Tarali, a woman I interviewed in 2004, was in grade 8 in Koroba High School, some young men broke into the girls' dormitory and raped her and a few other female students. Tarali became pregnant as a result and dropped out. In fact, Tarali knew the young man who had raped her, and she asserted that he had targeted her specifically because he hoped to force a marriage between them. He was trying to kill two birds with one stone, as it were. He was, with his gang, vandalizing the school and harming its students in order to express anger about the school's failure to pay sufficient compensation to the nearby community for the land it was occupying, but he was simultaneously trying to acquire a desired spouse who would otherwise have been far beyond his reach. He hoped that her parents would see their union as a solution to the problem of the premarital sex that he had forced upon her. As Tarali explained:

> The young man who raped me said that he knew I was a good young woman who did well in school and could marry an important, well-educated man, and so he chose me. [He knew you?] Yes, he knew me. . . . One of my sisters married a man from Koroba who lived very near the high school. He was her in-law. [So you knew him.] Yes, I knew him. We had stayed in the same house; we had eaten together. [So he knew you and he wanted to rape you?] Yes, he intended to rape me specifically. . . . My bed was in a room far from the door, and he deliberately came and looked for me. He chose me because he wanted to marry me. . . . But I didn't want to marry a man like him with no education. And I didn't want to marry someone who broke into the dorm and raped me.

Tarali was lucky: her family did not force her to marry her rapist, and when I interviewed her she was very happily married to a man she met a few years later. However, eight of the twenty-five women I interviewed in 2004 (including Tarali) were raped, five of them were forced to marry their rapists, and none of these marriages were happy.

Compensation Claims and Forensic Exams

The sexual violence during this period also led to a form of medical violence. While inquiring about the details of two village court cases concerning sexual assault (Tabitha and Madeline, discussed below), I learned about an unexpected development at the hospital: procedures for handling sexual assault patients had recently been created in order to meet demands for evidence in village court cases. Rape cases were being medicalized in the sense that victims were being brought to the hospital, when in the past they had not been unless they suffered additional injuries (e.g., broken bones, stab wounds). However, the medical treatment they received was not therapeutic. Rather, it was forensic, and forensically very specific to Huli concerns about premarital sex. In cases involving young unmarried female victims, the accused perpetrators had begun demanding that the victims be medically examined to determine (1) whether or not the young woman had been a virgin before the alleged assault, and (2) whether the alleged sex had been consensual or forced. Sometimes these examinations took place weeks after the incidents in question, since it often took that long for an incident to come to light, for the woman's kin to demand compensation, for a village court case to be scheduled, and for the alleged perpetrator's kin to respond by demanding the medical examination. Hospital staff either did not know that medical examinations cannot definitively answer the above questions, especially days or weeks after the event, or chose to proceed anyway, and thus the hospital records dutifully contained carbon copies of numerous letters like this one:

> F/16. The above named has been examined . . . one week later from the time she alleges she was raped by somebody (a man). She says this was the first time she had sexual intercourse. She was menstruating at the time of this incident. A young girl of about 16–17 years of age. Not in distress, no signs of scratches or wounds to the private parts—vulva is normal and vagina open. Adult speculum easily introduced in the vagina. My two fingers introduced as if she is far experienced with sex. No signs of healing lacerations of the introitus or posterior part of the vagina. And therefore not a virgin at all.

In other words, the medical finding in this case, documented in a letter purchased for use by the perpetrator, was that, contrary to her assertion, the girl had not been a virgin before the alleged rape and that it was possible that her rape claim was also false since there were no visible scratches, wounds, or lacerations. Impossible not to notice, as well, is the affective tone of moralistic judgment, and perhaps even pleasure, emerging from the text, despite its being encoded in seemingly objective, clinical language ("My two fingers introduced as if she is far experienced with sex. . . . And therefore not a virgin at all").

Setting aside the impossibility of reading facts about a woman's sexual history from a visual or tactile investigation of her vagina, it is important to understand how the "facts" produced from these exams were used. A young woman's kin hoped that an exam would show that she had been a virgin and that her claim of rape was true; this would enable them to demand a large compensation payment. The alleged perpetrator's kin were hoping for the opposite result: if it was determined that she had not been a virgin prior to the incident and that the sex had been consensual, then they could refuse to pay any compensation at all, arguing that she was a "loose" woman and that it was impossible to know how many previous partners she'd had. (This was the initial outcome in Tabitha's case, discussed below.) If a young woman was determined to have been a virgin, but the sex consensual, one or both parties might propose that the couple marry, in which case the alleged perpetrator's kin would pay bridewealth for her. In some ways the most contentious outcome was that a young woman was determined not to have been a virgin, but the incident was a rape. The evidence used to arrive at this outcome seemed to be that the girl's vaginal opening was large and smooth, the hymen was not intact and did not show any evidence of recent tearing, but there were other signs of forced sex such as lacerations on the vulva or injuries to other parts of the body. In this case, compensation could be demanded, but the man's kin would argue that it should be reduced because "someone else had stolen her first," and her family should therefore hunt down the earlier perpetrator(s) if they wanted full compensation for her "theft."

In general, Huli do not prize female virginity as valuable in and of itself, and it is not associated with some notion of female purity. Rather, it indexes a young woman's proper care, socialization, and discipline by her family; it is an indicator not just of her individual character, but of the character of her family and how they have raised her. As important, young women are said to begin experiencing sexual desire after they have first had sex, not before. By "opening up" a woman, penile penetration is said to initiate desire in her, and this desire should be initiated by and directed towards her husband. Much as Veena Das observes for Hindu society, drawing on Claude Lévi-Strauss's alliance theory, "A girl's awakening into sexuality is considered not as the work of her own desire but rather the working of male desire, which in the code of alliance is most appropriately the desire of her husband. The sexual offence of rape against a young girl thus becomes an offence against the code of alliance" (Das 1996: 2416). In other words, rape perverts the proper course of female desire and is thus a violation against men, both the men of her natal family who have rightful custody over her and the men who might want to marry her.

Das's analysis of judicial discourse in Indian court proceedings regarding rape suggested that judges' questioning often sought to determine "whether a body previously unmarked by the impress of male desire on it ha[d] been 'sexualised' through the offence under trial" (Das 1996: 2416)—that is, did the assault bring about a change in the girl or young woman such that she came to recognize herself as a sexual being. Similarly, Huli worry that a young woman whose desire has been "opened up" prior to marriage—including through rape—may find that usband is not enough for her, and it is thought that she is less likely to be faithful. The onset of female desire in this model has nothing to do with the pleasure or consensual nature of a woman's first sexual experience; rather, it is the physical penetration itself that is thought to produce desire. In conversations and during interviews, one of the concerns people articulated about the increase in sexual violence during this period was that it might result in more women becoming sex workers because of their excess desire.

Tabitha's Case

I never knew Tabitha. She was already dead when I arrived in 2004. She was the teenaged daughter of divorced parents, had gone to live with her father, and was raped by a young man in his household. The young man's kin insisted that she undergo a medical exam, and when the hospital report indicated that she had not been a virgin, they refused to pay compensation. Tabitha and her family were humiliated during the court case owing to the findings of the medical exam, and afterwards the young man's kin regularly insulted her in public, jeering at her pretensions that she, a *pamuk meri* (prostitute, slut), might get compensation from them. Tabitha committed suicide by hanging herself, and ultimately the young man's kin had to pay far more in compensation for her death than they would have if they had agreed to pay compensation for her rape, because their insults were deemed the primary *tene*—cause—of her suicide. Women's injuries to themselves, including suicide, are often a tactic of last resort for asserting the truth of their testimonies (Wardlow 1996, 2006a), and Tabitha's suicide was understood in this way, at least by most people I spoke with.

One wonders, of course, how the village court case (and perhaps Tabitha's life) might have proceeded differently in the absence of the damning forensic report. The report served to establish physical, historical, and moral "facts" about Tabitha that played a pivotal role in her suicide. In the past, village court cases did not always establish "the truth" of an event; sometimes they did, but sometimes they instead produced a sufficiently acceptable outcome in terms of an agreed amount for compensation that "the truth" of a matter could remain indeterminate. People might continue to grumble about the meaning of the events in question, but the dispute itself was resolved. One thing these forensic vaginal exams did, for the short period they existed, was assert the possibility and preeminence of a scientifically verified and unassailable truth (though they weren't, in fact, scientific, and could not produce truth). Arguably this made young women's testimony even less valuable, less worth listening to (cf. Mulla 2014). Nevertheless, Tabitha's suicide, as its own kind of unassailable truth, did, at least for some people, work to overturn the preeminence of the forensic exam as a signifier of a vagina's history, and thus also a signifier of a young woman's morality.

In the South African context, Elizabeth Thornberry (2015) has similarly argued that a change in practices for conducting virginity examinations among the Xhosa during the colonial period disempowered and silenced women. Precolonially, elderly female kin had the authority to examine young women in response to allegations of rape or premarital sex, but colonial courts demanded that medically trained doctors carry out these exams, thus eliminating older women's generational authority, as well as their practiced knowledge, in making these assessments. Whereas older female kin's findings generally accorded with a young woman's statement about a sexual incident, the focus on bodily evidence in medical exams meant that young women's testimony carried far less weight: only 25 percent of rape cases resulted in a verdict of guilty, Thornberry found. Virginity exams are not a Huli custom; nevertheless, the privileging of medical evidence over female testimony had a similar silencing effect, as Madeline's case demonstrates.

Madeline's Case

Madeline, a teenager, had been travelling with her parents and younger sister to a funeral when *rascals* (criminals) held up their PMV. While Madeline's mother and sister huddled near their father, Madeline had run into the forest, and when she returned, she claimed that one of the rascals had run after her and raped her. The alleged perpetrator was identified and compensation was demanded from his family, who demanded that Madeline undergo a medical exam. The resulting report stated that Madeline was pregnant, that she had not been a virgin before the attack, that it was possible that a rape had taken place, but also possible that the pregnancy was not due to the rape. The alleged perpetrator said that he had chased Madeline into the trees, but that he had not had sex with her. Female friends of Madeline were badgered into admitting that she had a boyfriend. Madeline herself was then repeatedly pestered by her female kin to reveal the truth of the situation: had she had sex with her boyfriend? Had she known she was pregnant before the attack? Had the accused actually attacked her, or was her story about what happened during the holdup a fabrication?

During one of these interrogations, at which I was present, a few women who had themselves been victims of a PMV holdup exchanged looks and noted dryly that Madeline's behavior had been aberrant: a young girl like her would have clung to her father, as her mother and sister had done, not run off into the bush on her own. The insinuation was that even as the attack was taking place, Madeline—unnaturally, disturbingly—had the presence of mind to spot the serendipitous opportunity: she could hide her premarital sexual dalliance by claiming she'd been raped during the holdup. A pregnancy due to rape was less stigmatizing than a pregnancy due to consensual premarital sex, because in the former she was an innocent victim, whereas in the latter case, she could be construed as "loose." Perhaps Madeline had calculated that if she ran into the bush, where there were no witnesses, no one would be the wiser.

Later that same day, when Madeline was absent, the women recalled their own experiences of being victims of a PMV holdup and gang rape the year before—their terror, the gasping for breath, their legs that suddenly went weak and wobbly. To ease the moment of painful recollection—a moment in which they were re-embodying the event, with one woman gulping for breath and another in tears—they teased each other. "I remember seeing you lose your footing and roll down the hill. Your skirt was up over your head and your petticoats were in the air. You looked like a fat chicken tumbling down that hill."[7] "And do you remember —? She was trying to whack that rascal with her umbrella." Ultimately, however, they drew on their own harrowing memories to analyze Madeline's account of her incident, and to agree that it raised troubling questions. Why had she not been paralyzed with fear, as they had been? How had she been able to run when they could barely breathe or coordinate their limbs? That Madeline's response to sexual violence had not been the same as theirs made them suspicious, which suggests that trauma can have the troubling impact on its survivors of making them doubt or even disqualify victims whose affective responses do not match their own.

Notably, all this speculation about Madeline's aberrant behavior and possible canny manipulation of events was voiced only *after* the results of her vaginal exam were made known. Until that moment, Madeline's female kin had forcefully upheld her version. In other words, the "factual" findings of the exam not only undermined her narrative, but also sowed doubts among those who would normally have zealously supported her.

It was at this point that Madeline suddenly refused to speak about the incident at all. In response to questions before, during, and after the village court case, she remained silent, head down, face studiously blank. She was also silent about the outcome, which was that the village court case against the alleged rapist was dropped, as were attempts to demand compensation from her supposed boyfriend. Both young men maintained that they had not had sex with her, and in the face of Madeline's silence and uncertain medical exam results, it became impossible to move forward litigiously. In the cases I knew about, the forensic exam silenced young women: Madeline went mute when she realized her kin might believe the exam over her own testimony. As Laura Hengehold has observed in the North American context, rape trials, with their requirements that victims' testimony correspond to preconceived narratives, can "turn [women's] desiring and discursive energies against themselves when they attempt to describe 'what happened'" (Hengehold 2000: 193). Madeline, with her vagina appropriated from her by the forensic exam and used to contradict her voice, chose silence. However, it also seemed that her resolute silence had powerful social effects: her refusal to cooperate, explain, justify, or make herself legible to others ultimately derailed their attempts to create and resolve a dispute about her sexual conduct.

A conjunction of factors drove this intimate forensic scopic economy in which a girl or young woman was re-violated in order to reveal "facts" that would enable a dispute to be resolved and compensation paid or withheld. There was, of course, the widespread sexual violence during this period, which resulted in an increase in compensation claims. Not to demand compensation was shameful, and was read as a family's disavowal of the woman, a decision that she was not worth pursuing redress. Moreover, if compensation wasn't demanded, there was the possibility that a girl's "brothers" (whether natal or more broadly defined male kin) would take matters into their own hands and rape "sisters" of the alleged perpetrator, or otherwise take revenge, dangerously escalating a conflict. Concurrent with an increase in sexual violence, however, there was also concern about increases in consensual premarital sex, with many people asserting that young women were "no longer fenced in"—that is, not as well monitored and controlled as in the past. Thus, when a woman's kin alleged rape, a young man's kin was likely to allege consent. It was hoped that medical evidence could resolve this kind of impasse. Finally, over time there has been a more general escalation in the demands for medical evidence in Huli compensation cases. Where testimony, witness confirmation, or community knowledge about complainant and accused had been sufficient in the past, now medical documentation had become part of the assemblage of making grievances visible and compensable (see also van Amstel and van der Geest 2004).

Alice Street has argued that in Papua New Guinea, X-rays and other visibilizing health technologies might better be considered "relational technologies," rather than biopolitical or even diagnostic technologies, because their importance for patients is not that they "could now know and see what was inside them but that, in being rendered recognizable and knowable within the conventions of biomedicine . . . doctors would feel compelled to cure them" (Street 2014: 131). In other words, from a patient's perspective, particularly in a context of scarce medical resources, the X-ray is less about revealing the truth of the body and more about being able to produce oneself as the kind of person—a patient—who can solicit therapeutic attention from the busy doctor, whose presence and care are perpetually elsewhere. Any assumption that Tari Hospital's forensic vaginal exams had biopolitical or medicalizing effects is similarly problematic, though in this case, the visualizing technology might better be thought of as a *moral* technology rather than a relational one. Through attempting to use the exams to visibilize morality within the vagina, the exam worked to produce young women as particular kinds of female persons: prior virgins whose injuries could compel compensation from others or, more often than not, according to the records I examined, "far experienced with sex" and thus unable to be recognized as worthy compensable subjects. Governmental abandon meant that there was no oversight of hospital practice and thus nothing to prevent the development of this anomalous procedure. What gave these exams their authority and scientific truth-value was the fact that they were carried out in the state-authorized site of the hospital, using state-trained employees and state-provided equipment. However, this was unsanctioned practice that emerged in the vacuum created by the state's absence.[8] These exams quickly disappeared once order in Tari was restored.

TRANSACTIONAL SEX

Passenger Women

Last Minute Lucy was sometimes meanly teased by family members for "catching AIDS at the last minute," by which they meant at a later stage in life, when most people assume a woman's sexual activity is winding down or over. Wearing big hoop earrings and a colorful skirt, she looked to be in her early fifties when I first interviewed her in 2012. She was living with her younger brother, who was also HIV-positive, and they were another of the nuclear family clusters that made me concerned that HIV prevalence in the Tari area was significantly higher than the reported national prevalence. They had not spent much time together after their youth—indeed, had lived in different provinces for most of their adulthood. In other words, they did not belong to the same sexual networks, which might have resulted in them both being infected. They were living together when I interviewed Lucy because neither was married and both had been ostracized by their other siblings because of their HIV-positive status.

Lucy said she'd had a disastrous marriage when she was much younger. Her husband had infected her repeatedly with gonorrhea, often refused to go to the hospital to be tested or treated, and was later convicted of raping a young girl and was sent to prison. "After that I'd had enough," she said. "That was enough of marriage for me. I decided to live alone. He'd fucked around and ruined that girl and ruined my life, so I decided I would passenger around too. I went around and was friends with lots of men."

She soon tired of this lifestyle, however, and moved into her older brother's household. According to her, she hadn't had sex for forty years. Given my estimation of her age, this did not seem likely, and I understood this statement as signifying both a very long time and, with its possible gesture towards the Israelites wandering in the wilderness, a kind of self-imposed penance for her earlier unrestrained ways. Dependent on her older brother for land and a home, she had dutifully cooked and cleaned for his household.

> And then, at the last minute, my brother hit me. [Why?] He didn't like the way I'd prepared his dinner. I'd been caring for his household for years, and then one night he lost his temper about having to eat sweet potato all the time, and he hit me. So I left. I decided to passenger around again. I went to a *dawe anda*, I befriended a man, I went home with him, and I caught AIDS.

To "passenger around" is a euphemism for sleeping around, and "passenger women" are women who have abandoned home and family with the intent of having extramarital sexual relationships, often in exchange for money (Wardlow 2002, 2004, 2006a). Like Lucy, they sometimes assert that relationships in which they felt unjustly and poorly treated triggered their decision to take this step. Some simply want to escape a situation they find intolerable, and some describe their actions as a kind of revenge promiscuity—that is, they flagrantly engage in inappropriate sexual conduct in order to anger and shame those who have wronged them. Last Minute Lucy described two periods of her life when anger drove her to become a "passenger woman." The first was in response to her husband's philandering and her inability to protect herself from repeated sexually transmitted infections. Her infertility, likely caused by these repeated infections, his sexual assault of a child, and her consequent rage and humiliation motivated her to set off on her own and befriend men as necessary. Much later in her life, feeling unappreciated by her older brother and wrongly beaten by him, she again set off on her own, this time heading straight for a *dawe anda*. *Dawe anda* are secluded houses somewhat like brothels, where men sing traditional courtship songs to the women there and sometimes pay them for sex (Wardlow 2006a: 193–95). Three other women in my sample of thirty women living with HIV also said that they'd left their households in anger—because of a husband's infidelities or his violence—and decided to "passenger around." They did not know whether they had been infected by their husbands or by their subsequent sexual partners.

By 2004, the term "passenger woman" (*pasinja meri* in Tok Pisin, *pasinja wali* in Huli) seemed to be falling out of usage in Tari, and the descriptor *pasinja* had changed somewhat in meaning compared to the mid 1990s when I had done my doctoral research. People had begun referring to some men as *pasinja man* and groups of people as *pasinja manmeri*. These latter usages referred to men or people who drank, gambled, and often traveled from one place to another looking for opportunities to engage in these activities. They would hear about a lively *dawe anda* and go there for a while, and then move on to the next diversion. They were described as lazy, irresponsible, and unwilling to undertake the hard work of caring for a family. Passenger women were, in addition, assumed to sell sex or otherwise engage in inappropriate liaisons.

Notably, in 2004, passenger women did not seem to be any more vilified for their behavior than passenger men. Moreover, despite the widespread sexual violence in the mid 2000s, I heard of no cases that were specifically about punishing passenger women for their sexual behavior. This was a profound departure from the mid 1990s, when most of the violent sexual assaults I heard about were said to be of passenger women who deserved what they got simply because they were passenger women. In the 1990s, a woman's embrace of sexual autonomy, and especially her sale of sex, were seen by some as so profoundly wrong and threatening to the social order that she might be gang-raped or murdered (cf. Moffett 2006). The intense rancor that animated these ideas had diminished by the mid 2000s. Selling sex was still considered immoral; however, the degree of animosity towards women who did so had lessened significantly. This shift should be understood in the context of Tari's socioeconomic decline in the late 1990s and early 2000s. Most important, I think, was the evaporation of ways for women to make money, a situation that made many people take a more generous attitude towards women who sold sex "for the right reasons" (e.g., to pay children's school fees).

The Rise of Transactional Sex

As discussed above, during this period, many stores and government offices closed, resulting in the loss of employment for those in less-skilled jobs (e.g., clerks, cleaners), some of whom were women. More important for most women was the flight of civil servants, health workers, and teachers. Many rural women make their money by selling produce and other items (betel nut, loose cigarettes, etc.) to the employed, and with many of the employed having fled the area, and the remainder unable to access their pay, women had far fewer customers for their goods. Men still had some means of making money, however. A number were employed by PJV, for example, and there was eventually an influx of police—both regular and mobile squad (all men at that time). And the hospital and the few remaining stores all had male security guards. Given this situation of female economic precarity, it is perhaps not surprising that the number of women selling sex increased. As one man said, "We would have to blindfold ourselves not to see all the willing women here now."

Moreover, with more women selling sex, the price to buy it plummeted (Wardlow 2007, 2009). Many of the men interviewed by my male field assistants in 2004 commented on how easy it had become to find a woman who was willing to have sex for a small amount of money—approximately two dollars, compared with approximately twelve dollars in the mid 1990s. In the 1990s, only some men could afford this higher price, and the ability to buy sex was a marker of inequality between men. Indeed, my impression at that time was that some men's condemnation of passenger women stemmed more from their resentment at not being able to afford them than from a feeling of moral offense. In contrast, in 2004, with lower prices, buying sex was no longer a source of division between men and instead became a means for them to solidify their camaraderie. Now that more men could partake, more men could share stories and compare notes, as suggested by an interview one of my field assistants did with a married man, who said:

> I get very graphic when I talk about passenger women. I say, "This woman is willing to do this or that." Or, "Her genitals looked like this." Or, "That woman's genitals feel like that." My friends are the same—they boast about the different styles they've tried. They say, "She was in this position and I did this," or "I pushed her down and did it to her like that." We really talk about sex and passenger women in a very explicit way. And when one man does this, it gives the rest of us the idea to try a particular style or try a particular woman.

Moreover, my later research in 2012 and 2013 suggested that warfare, emotional trauma, male solidarity, and sexual risk were complexly intertwined. Some men I spoke with at the AIDS Care Centre said that after they'd fled their own territory due to tribal fighting, they had been taken in by male kin who had encouraged them to attend *dawe anda* and had paid their entrance fees. As mentioned earlier, *dawe anda* (literally, courtship houses) are enclosed sites where men can gather to form teams and compete for women's attention by singing traditional erotic courtship songs. The women who attend are typically there to sell sex (though if they are divorced or widowed, they may also be hoping to find a new husband). In public discourse *dawe anda* are stigmatized as places of illicit sexual transaction: "good women" do not attend, and young unmarried men, whose bodies are said to be easily polluted by sex, are not supposed to. The men at the AIDS Care Centre who had been forced to flee their homes said that the ebullient and boisterous male fellowship, the flirtatious banter with women, the singing of *dawe anda* songs, and the sex all helped to dissipate feelings of terror and loss.

More generally, during this difficult period, many people knew women whom they thought of as "good women"—that is, women known to be hardworking, respectful, and generous—who had exchanged sex for money in order to buy food or pay their children's school fees. The fact that many more women were selling sex seemed to produce not only an alarmist response, but also a more nuanced, and often generous, parsing of sex sellers' moral characters. For example, some of my female friends, who in the past had condemned passenger women, suggested that women who sold sex occasionally out of economic need shouldn't really be thought of as passenger women or *pamuk meri* (sex workers). They associated these terms with women who gambled, drank, abandoned their children, and were "in the pocket of one man one day and another the next." To their minds the terms "passenger women" and *pamuk meri* failed to capture the challenging situations and moral decision-making of the women they knew. In short, aware of Tari's dire situation, and experiencing its miseries themselves, many people seemed to accept that necessity might drive some women to regrettable but not condemnable sexual behavior.

CONCLUSION

In Papua New Guinea, where the lack of infrastructure and services is perpetually lamented, people express an acute "desire for the state," Alice Street observes (2012: 1), and they often work assiduously to gain visibility in its eyes. People living in the Hela region during this period experienced, not just disregard by the state, but state abandonment—that is, the refusal of the state to "see" a populace, the withdrawal of its recognition. The violent and coercive sexual relations that emerged should not be seen as a reversion to brutal cultural tradition, which is how violence in Hela is often represented in Papua New Guinean newspapers, and more recently, in social media. Rather, state abandonment produced fear, anger, frustration, and desperation. It also enabled a vicious cycle of post-election clan conflict and crime to spiral out of control.

It is important to note that the cascading consequences of state abandonment accentuated gender asymmetries and vulnerabilities. Many of ways that rural Papua New Guinean women make money (e.g., selling produce or chickens) all but disappeared when government employees fled or could no longer access their wages. Not surprisingly, some women turned to transacting sex in order to gain cash for school fees and basic store goods, such as rice or cooking oil. And as the policing and court systems became dysfunctional, families came to rely on their young men for protection and intimidation of enemies; sexual violence was a tool in their arsenal. State abandonment also resulted in a form of medical violence against young women: spurious virginity exams that were used to resolve disputes about the compensability of alleged sexual assaults. Finally, crime—complexly entangled with clan conflicts—increased, and when PMVs or private vehicles were held up by armed gangs, rape of the female passengers was common. HIV vulnerability was therefore not simply a matter of whether women had the power to refuse sex or demand condom use. Rather, as this chapter demonstrates, HIV vulnerability is a question of how sexual interactions—desired, coerced, or forced—are shaped in the crucible of specific political histories.

3

Love, Polygyny, and HIV

Miriam met her first husband in 1991 when she was returning home to Tari, after having lived in Mt. Hagen with her uncle's family for almost two years. As she recalled, there had been tribal fighting along the road, and the area was unnaturally quiet. A number of bridges had been sabotaged, forcing Miriam and her uncle to leave their PMV and walk the rest of the way. The man who was to become her husband, armed and dressed as a warrior, offered to help carry their bags and accompany them safely through the conflict zone. Thereafter she repeatedly ran into him and his sister in Tari, and they would all walk around town together. Before they married, "He would boss me around (*Em save bossim mi*)," she said matter-of-factly, without resentment. "He would say, 'You can't go into Tari all the time.' He would say that he was going to marry me, and so I had to stay at home." (The implication here is that young women go into town to make themselves visible to potential suitors, and so if she continued to go to Tari, she would have been presenting herself as still available for marriage.)

The 2004 interview protocol included the question, "Can you tell me about a time when you were married and your husband did something that made you really happy?" Most women responded with stories about receiving gifts of money or clothing, or being praised or appreciated by a husband in front of his family. In contrast, Miriam told me about the time he introduced her to mutual oral sex. As she described it, they had been washing clothes on a beautiful day at a small, remote waterfall. "He just about died—he expressed so much pleasure. And he said things to me like, 'Oh Miriam, my love, this is too much. I am dying!' And I felt the same way, and we both finished our worries (*pinisim wari bilong mipela*, a euphemism for orgasm). We were really joined. . . . I still think about the sex we had together. It really joined us. What we did together was against Huli custom (*brukim lo bilong mipela*), and I don't think that other Huli spouses do the things we did together. We were really joined."

When Miriam states that oral sex is "against Huli custom," she is referring to the traditional ethic of gender avoidance, in which husbands and wives lived in different houses, cooked and ate separately, and generally conducted their lives in separate spheres. This ethic of distance was also supposed to inform marital sexual practice: sex was supposed to take place only a few days each month and only genital-to-genital sex was condoned. Some older male interviewees also spoke of lifting themselves up on their forearms to minimize bodily contact, or of rubbing a special red tree oil on their bellies and thighs before sex as a kind of protective barrier. These spatio-sexual distancing practices were intended to preserve a man's health, youthful vigor, martial strength, and social appeal.

Marriage has changed significantly since the pre- and early postcolonial period; nevertheless, only a few women in my 2004 interview sample spoke of having oral sex with their husbands, and all of them, like Miriam, described this as "against custom," "unnatural" (because not aimed at reproduction), "white" (because seen in pornographic magazines and films in which the performers were white), and something only sex workers did. While a husband was entitled to sex because he had paid bridewealth, women said, he wasn't entitled to *that kind* of sex; rather, he was entitled to reproduction-oriented sex. Most men in the sample, though not all, said that they engaged in "customary sex" with their wives, and that passenger women were for experimenting with "style-style sex," thus reinforcing the notion that sex with wives was for reproduction and that only rebellious and dissolute women engaged in non-customary sex. Some men also asserted that a man was asking for trouble if he introduced his wife to new sexual positions and practices: she might be more likely to seek out pleasure elsewhere, and, knowledgeable about his own predilections, she would be better able to manipulate and dominate him (Wardlow 2008). Some also worried that in anger a wife might publicly announce a husband's non-traditional sexual proclivities in order to humiliate him. In short, the 2004 interviews suggested that sexual practices that were perceived as "non-traditional" could complicate marital relations of power by introducing new emotional and psychological vulnerabilities into marriage. They were therefore to be avoided. One important consequence was that wives like Miriam, who did engage in non-customary practices, often felt that they had achieved a special and rare degree of intimacy, shared understanding, and trust in their marriages that other couples did not have. As Miriam put it, "We had secret pleasures together—we did things that other people don't know about. So we were really joined."

Miriam's husband worked as a coffee buyer, and he used some of his profits to set up a small trade store in Tari, which he trusted Miriam to manage when he was away. His willingness to leave her in charge of their store, and her sense that they were striving as a team for upward mobility, further reinforced Miriam's confidence and joy in having a real partnership with her husband.

It came as a complete shock to her, then, when without warning or discussion, he took a second wife. He had slept with other women before, she knew, and, in fact, she had once caught him in the act and "poked" his sexual partner with a knife (Huli women use the verb *pokim* to mean a light stab that draws blood, and might require stitches, but does not result in life-threatening injuries). However, he explained his sexual dalliances as meaningless stopgap measures made necessary because of his and Miriam's adherence to pregnancy and post-partum sexual abstinence rules, an explanation she accepted. Surreptitiously assembling bridewealth and taking another wife was another matter entirely.

Feeling profoundly betrayed, Miriam reacted by *bekim bek* (to get back at someone, to retaliate by engaging in equivalent hurtful behavior, usually used by Huli women to refer to revenge sex): "I was really angry with my husband, and so I went and had sex with another man. But my father found out, and he hit me and broke my nose, and then he told my husband." Her husband demanded a divorce and the return of all twenty-four of his bridewealth pigs. Because Miriam had given him three children, in the end he only received eight pigs, plus an additional seven from Miriam's sexual partner as compensation for the adultery.

Miriam was despondent after the demise of this marriage. She had expected that her infidelity might result in a physical altercation with her husband, but that he would eventually understand and forgive the rage that had driven her retaliatory behavior: "We were really joined. It should have been hard to rip us apart, hard to make him kick me out." But she had underestimated the anger he would feel at being humiliated by her infidelity and at her unwillingness to accept that, as a man, he had a right to take another wife, and, as a successful businessman, of course he had done so.

"So after that I just passengered around. I slept around with a lot of men. I went to *dawe anda*. I drank beer. I slept anywhere in any house." She lived for a while in Mt. Hagen, where a female cousin acted as a kind of sexual intermediary, informing her about men who were interested in her, and then taking a share of the money she made. Eventually, she moved back to Tari, traveled from one *dawe anda* to another, and met the man who became her second husband: "At one *dawe anda*, I was playing cards and a man came and sat behind me and gave me tips, told me what cards to play. And I won, so I gave him ten kina. And right then and there he announced that I was his wife. So I went home with him, and I've been with him for three years."

This "husband" had not given bridewealth for her, however, and he continued to attend *dawe anda*, where he occasionally had sex with other women:

> I know he has sex with other women, so I don't trust him, and it's hard for us to have private thoughts together. My first husband—it was like we had one name, one thought (*wanpela nem, wanpela tingting*; this could also be translated as having the same name, the same thought or way of thinking). But my thoughts are not joined with my second husband. I have wanted to teach him about the sexual things I did with my first husband, but I can't trust him. If I taught him he might go try them with other women, experience all kinds of pleasure with them, and then leave me altogether.

Notice here Miriam's assumptions that her second husband doesn't already know about non-customary sexual practices and that experiencing them would dramatically transform his relationship to his own desiring body. These assumptions speak, I think, to the pleasure, danger, and secrecy that Huli, perhaps especially women, associated with non-reproductive sex at that time.

. . .

Of the thirty HIV-positive women I interviewed in 2012 and 2013, at least twenty-two had been infected with HIV by their husbands. (Three more had been married to men who were also HIV-positive and who had histories of extramarital partners. Upon learning of their husband's infidelities, these women, much like Miriam, had *bekim bek,* and they did not know if they had contracted HIV from their husbands or from their subsequent partners.) Clearly, marriage is a site of HIV vulnerability, and the directionality of transmission is most often from husbands to wives. It is therefore important to understand how HIV vulnerability is produced within marriage, and Miriam's story introduces a number of important themes. For example, as a successful coffee buyer who had disposable income and was often away from home, Miriam's husband in fact had many extramarital partners (she learned of this after the dissolution of her marriage). Moreover, his polygyny also contributed to her HIV vulnerability, not, in this case, by introducing a new sexual partner into the marriage, but rather by betraying the kind of marriage Miriam thought they had, and thereby motivating her to engage in revenge sex. Her later depression, and her means of expressing and coping with it through a physically and sexually vagabond existence, can also be attributed to the demise of this marriage. And the demise of this marriage ultimately resulted from her and her husband's conflicting ideas about the nature of their marriage. They did not, in fact, have *wanpela tingting* when it came to polygyny, for example. In other words, marriage is a site of HIV vulnerability in part because Huli men and women often have very different and conflicting aspirations for marriage, and when these opposing desires and assumptions collide, it can result in either or both spouses seeking out extramarital partners.

AIDS PREVENTION AND THE PROMOTION
OF COMPANIONATE MARRIAGE

It is also important to examine marriage as a site of HIV vulnerability because AIDS prevention in the Tari area has focused not only on urging couples to "Be faithful"—the B of so-called ABC campaigns—but also on trying to teach them what loving, equitable, and health-promoting marriages should look like. For example, Population Services International (PSI) has developed and carries out four-day marital relationship training workshops for married couples in Hela that aim to equip them with a range of skills: active listening, using "I-statements" instead of "You-statements,"[1] understanding the concepts of intimacy and empathy and how to increase them, goal-setting for couples, and conflict de-escalation.[2] Marital relations in Papua New Guinea are often represented in the HIV/AIDS policy literature as pathogenic (see also Shih et al. 2017), and AIDS education, as well as gender-based violence reduction initiatives, have been animated by what might be called, borrowing from Tania Li (2007), a "will to improve" marital intimacy. Much as Anne Esacove observes, "policy prescribes and ultimately attempts to create 'modern' relationships as the solution to HIV/AIDS. . . . Reaching this prescriptive ideal requires a reorganization of intimate relationships" (Esacove 2016). Such interventions draw on a therapeutic ethos (Spronk 2009) and are often informed by a tacit evolutionist teleology of intimacy in which AIDS (and gender-based violence) might be prevented if people could learn to do heterosexual marriage in more modern, Western ways.

The marital model being promoted and taught in such workshops is often referred to in the social science literature as companionate marriage—that is, marriage in which "emotional closeness is understood to be both one of the primary measures of success in marriage and a central practice through which the relationship is constituted and reinforced" (Wardlow and Hirsch 2006: 4). The theorization of companionate marriage is often traced back to Anthony Giddens's 1992 book *The Transformation of Intimacy: Sexuality, Love, and Eroticism in Modern Societies,* in which he argued that "modern societies"—by which he meant Western, or Northern, societies—had undergone a significant constellation of social, economic, and ideological changes, such that romantic love, or what he called a "pure relationship," had achieved a kind of ascendency and had become the precursor to, and foundation for, intimate relationships like marriage. A pure relationship, he said, is created and sustained by sentiment—the self's emotional fulfillment by the other's unique qualities. With sentiment at its core, companionate marriage can be distinguished from marital forms in which, for example, political or economic alliances between families are prioritized.

Although it is being promoted in Papua New Guinea, it is important to note that feminist and queer theorists have advanced important critiques of this marital form. Scholars have observed, for example, that the valorization of companionate marriage is a fundamental component of a modern heteronormative narrative that also includes the assumption that monogamous intimacy between two people is the one and only path to happiness (Berlant 1998, Ahmed 2010, Wilson 2012). As Lauren Berlant puts it, "desires for intimacy that bypass the couple or the life narrative it generates have no alternative plots"; "only one plot counts as 'life' (first comes love, then . . .)," and departing from the love-then-marriage-then-baby-carriage trajectory is viewed as not a real life: "Those who don't or can't find their way in that story—the queers, the single, the something else—can become so easily unimaginable, even often to themselves" (1998: 285–86). Sara Ahmed, for her part, expresses skepticism about "the happiness turn" (Ahmed 2010: 3) and the centrality of companionate marriage to it. What she calls the happiness turn refers to the recent global wholesale cultural embrace of happiness as that which "gives purpose, meaning and order to human life" (1), so that there are now global surveys, academic journals, and an enormous therapeutic industry devoted to measuring, analyzing, and promoting happiness and the ways to achieve it. She notes that "one of the primary happiness indicators is marriage" (6), and she traces the ways that "happiness promotion becomes very quickly the promotion of certain types of families" (11). In other words, the promise and hegemonic value of happiness legitimates the normalization of families founded on companionate marriage, and the delegitimation of other forms of intimacy. Finally, anthropologists have pointed out the fragility of marital forms based on happy, gratifying sentiment: if the marriage ceases to produce happiness, it can be dissolved, with sometimes devastating consequences for women, who are often dependent on husbands, both economically and, in some contexts, reputationally (Wardlow and Hirsch 2006).

It is important to note that the globalization of companionate conjugality as happiness-producing, or "the only plot," works to exclude or delegitimize not only queer intimacies, but also other non-Western/Northern forms of heterosexual intimacy. The heteronormative conjugal couple assumed by critiques such as Berlant's and Ahmed's is a Western/Northern one. In contrast, while the Huli might also be considered strongly heteronormative, their precolonial philosophies and practices regarding conjugality do not accord with the companionate models of marriage promulgated in Papua New Guinea by Christian churches, state institutions, or, more recently, AIDS education programming. Central to the companionate marriage model promoted by these various institutions is the idea that "real" intimacy is what might be called *proximate intimacy*, in which affective closeness between spouses is achieved through living together, face-to-face communication, shared activities, and the mutual disclosure of the vulnerable emotional self to the conjugal other. Miriam's words expressed it well: "it was like we had one name, one thought."

In contrast, precolonial Huli philosophies about marriage and marital intimacy were underpinned by an ethic of what I call *distant intimacy*—intimacy achieved and sustained by *avoiding* excessive psychological and spatial closeness. Huli men tend to feel that distant intimacy is a better way of doing marriage, while Huli women tend to aspire to making their marriages more companionate. Women associate companionate marriage not only with emotional attachment between spouses, but also with true friendship between them, equal (or almost equal) participation in household decision-making, greater loyalty to each other rather than to their natal families, sexual fidelity, and monogamy (as opposed to polygyny). They also view it as offering them important practical benefits, such as being able to exert more influence over a husband and his resources. And while some men crave and appreciate proximate intimacy with their wives, many also associate it with the loss of male autonomy and privilege. One way to think about the recent history of marriage among the Huli, then, is as a story about a contested, ambivalent, fitful, and sometimes violent shift from distant intimacy towards proximate intimacy.

PROXIMATE INTIMACY AND DISTANT INTIMACY

Of all the narratives I have collected about Huli marriages from 2004 to 2013, Miriam's is the one that most aligns with the companionate marriage model, particularly in terms of emotional closeness being at its center (at least as this marriage was experienced by her; her husband may or may not have had this same affective experience). This emotional intimacy was achieved and reinforced in a number of ways: through choosing each other, living in the same house, sleeping in the same room, conversing pleasurably with each other, building businesses together, and engaging in what she experienced as adventurous and mutually gratifying sex.

As noted above, this model represents a profound departure from precolonial and early postcolonial marital philosophies and practices. Participants in my 2004 research were asked to describe the structure and composition of their childhood household, and to compare it to their own marital household. Twenty-two of the twenty-five women I interviewed said that their fathers and mothers had lived in separate houses, sometimes even on different clan territories, and many said that they rarely saw their fathers when they were children. In contrast, twenty-three of the twenty-five women lived with their husbands and children in one house, representing a dramatic change in household structure over just one generation. Typical of their descriptions of their childhood households were statements like these:

> How my father lived or what he ate, I never knew. He had his own house and fields. . . . When my father wanted to talk to my mother, he would stand outside her house with his back to the door. He wouldn't look at her. He wouldn't go inside her house or even come close to it. He didn't stand face-to-face with her and talk to her. (Jessie)

> My father slept in his own house, and we didn't see him very often. We saw him when it was time to kill a pig for a feast or a compensation payment. At that time, men were men. Very different from now. They didn't sit around and talk with their wives and children, or joke around with them or play with them or do little things to make them happy, make them laugh. My husband isn't like that. He went to school, and he knows the new ways of doing things. He spends lots of time with our children and me. (Gabby)

The men interviewed in 2004 made very similar generational contrasts, though more of them expressed anger and resentment about rarely seeing their fathers, and they also attributed their fathers' absences to labor migration, and not only to there being separate residences for husbands and wives. Traditionally, sons are supposed to move out of their mother's house and into their father's house at about age ten, as a necessary stage in their transition to adult masculinity. They can't, of course, if a father isn't there, so it is perhaps not surprising that men felt a father's absence more acutely. What emerged from both men's and women's descriptions of their parents' marriages was a model of "distant intimacy" that was already, even when the participants were children, being frayed by male out-migration to work in mines and plantations in other provinces.

The practice of distant intimacy stems from the premise that a man's and his family's health, vitality, and social success depend on men and women, including spouses, eschewing too much corporeal contact. The ethnographic literature about Papua New Guinea often refers to this as "gender separation," and has emphasized men's avoidance or careful management of female substances—menstrual blood, in particular. I instead use the term "distant intimacy" in order to suggest that there may be ways of imagining and enacting attachments to and entanglements with cherished others that do not include constant physical, verbal, and emotional sharing. The men interviewed by my male field assistants in 2004 emphasized the powerful nature and potential danger not only of a wife's sexual fluids, but also of her talk, touch, smell, and breath (Wardlow 2008, 2014). Many asserted that spousal co-residence (living in the same house) caused premature aging in a man because of the mutual porosity of conjugally linked bodies and the consequent damaging effects of excessive intimacy. Breathing in a wife's exhaled breath, hearing her angry talk cut into one's body, inhaling smoke from a fire made from wood she might have stepped over (thereby contaminating it), —all these female bodily emanations were described as "substances" that could move out of a wife's body into her husband's, causing harm.

In addition to concerns about corporeal intrusions, many men worried about the ways in which conjugal co-residence enabled spouses to "know each other too well." To know one's spouse too well was to know his or her desires, emotional frailties, and past humiliations; it was thus to know exactly what to say to cause emotional injury (which was often described as phenomenologically feeling like a bodily injury). And although men most feared a wife's ability to inflict emotional damage in this way, they also spoke worriedly of the reverse—of being so angry that they used their intimate knowledge about a wife to inflict emotional pain upon her. In short, they expressed grave misgivings about proximate intimacy—the psychological closeness that is at the core of companionate marriage. One might be tempted to assume that such concerns are culturally specific to the Huli. However, it is worth considering that they may be inherent in companionate marriage itself. Analyzing "morbid companionate marriage" (i.e., unhappily married couples) in the United States, Candace Vogler notes that many of them were "mired in something like epistemic overkill"—"so profound a knowledge of their spouses' selves that they can silence or push them to the breaking point with the simplest of gestures" (Vogler 1998: 329–30). Such "epistemic overkill"— and its potentially injurious consequences—is exactly what Huli (more often men than women) were describing when they talked about the dangers of "knowing each other too well."

It is impossible to know how "distant intimacy" was subjectively experienced by married couples in the precolonial past, but today, gender separation is motivated by a range of emotions. For some, a selective and partial practice of gender avoidance can be a form of intimate mutual care, and not just a way for men to protect themselves from women's corporeal and affective incursions. The elderly man quoted below had been trained as a youth to rigorously follow gender separation practices, but at the time of the interview lived happily with his wife in the same house:

> I joined a school for *ibagiya* for almost two years when I was young. (*Ibagiya* are bachelors, and "schools" such as the one to which he refers are called "bachelor cults" in older ethnographic literature. They were intended to train young men in hunting, warfare, and practices for keeping their bodies healthy and pure.) If we broke the rules, the leaders could tell just by looking at our bodies. There was no way to hide from them. We weren't allowed to look at women or even walk on the same trails. We carried special leaves to wipe away women's footprints, and we recited special spells as we walked along to protect ourselves from the smell or footprints women might have left behind. . . . I still follow many of these rules: I never accept food from my wife when she's menstruating. We live in one house, but we sleep in separate rooms. We enjoy talking to each other and eating together, but she may not touch my belongings or go into my room. Living together makes us both happy.

Other elderly men and women who maintained the practice of separate marital residences spoke of how the giving of bridewealth joined spouses' bodies so that they became more sensorially attuned to each other, such that one might feel a spouse's illness or injury, even if living elsewhere. A few, for example, spoke of suddenly feeling pain or malaise, viscerally knowing that something was wrong with a spouse, and running to the spouse's house to find that he or she was sick or had been injured. Intimacy in these marriages was not about mutual psychological disclosure or the sharing of affectively laden talk, but rather about phenomenologically joined bodily experience (even across physical distance), mutual corporeal care (through separate bodily practices that nevertheless helped to ensure the other's health), and the vivid imagining of the spatially distant conjugal other.

Some men who had given proximate intimacy a try rejected it when they observed its impact on their marriage, which they often experienced as a loss of autonomy or dominance. For example, one 54-year-old man who'd had four wives said:

> Although I've seen blue movies (i.e., pornography), I haven't tried to do any of these things with my wives. I think the purpose of marital sex is to have children. This is our custom, and so I have sex the traditional way, with my wife on her back underneath me. Actually, my second wife liked to try different kinds of styles—when I asked her to try things I'd seen in blue movies or magazines, she agreed and she enjoyed it a lot. But I think this is why she became so rebellious and defiant. She liked it best when she was on top. . . . But then I noticed that my body was getting weaker and weaker. Also I noticed that she was becoming more demanding, and more likely

to get angry with me, and that she no longer showed me respect. So now I think all these different styles are bad. They are bad for marriage. I really wanted to try all these different things with her, but my desire for this made me confused, and she took advantage of me. So I divorced her.

In this case, mutual sexual pleasure and the proximate intimacy that comes from revealing one's sexual longings upended the customary norms of male dominance in marriage, leaving this man feeling threatened. Significantly, the corporeal and the structural are linked in this narrative, so that a wife's corporeal ascendancy during sex (being on top) becomes her structural ascendancy in the marriage, while the loss of male dominance manifests itself not only in the husband's loss of control over his wife's behavior, but also in his corporeal weakness.

Such concerns endure in the present, making men more skeptical and ambivalent about models of intimacy that might threaten male autonomy and dominance. One consequence is that men often seek out male-only or male-dominant spaces and activities (snooker houses, makeshift taverns, *dawe anda*) as a kind of antidote for too much time spent in contact with a wife.

BUILDING A COMPANIONATE MARRIAGE, AND THE BETRAYAL OF POLYGYNY

According to women who described their marital relations as companionate, their marriages were forged, not only through mutually pleasurable sex or intimate conversation, but also through feeling that they and their husbands were working together as a team for upward mobility. Miriam was proud, for example, that her husband trusted her to run their trade store when he was away: their relatively egalitarian economic partnership confirmed for her that their relationship was special. Helen's husband, who worked as a driver in the tourism industry, was able to get her a job as a hotel maid, and, although theirs had been an arranged marriage, they quickly became very emotionally close, a closeness that Helen attributed to the fact that they pooled their resources and decided together on significant purchases:

[Were you able to sit down and talk with your husband? Did you become friends?] Yes, we became friends. We would walk around town together, and go shopping together. When I was forced to marry him, I was unhappy and angry. But once we moved to —, and I was working and I had my own money, I was happy. He got me a job, so I was happy with him. And we saved some money to buy a block of land. We talked, we joked around. [What did you like to talk about?] We were happy when we would talk about saving our money and moving back to Tari to start a little business together. We would talk about the future—about saving money to buy chickens and start a little business.

Jessie, another woman I interviewed, similarly became very close to her husband through mutually pleasurable sex and joint egalitarian strategizing for upward mobility. Unlike Miriam's marriage, which was formed by choice, or Helen's marriage, which was arranged, Jessie's isn't easily categorized. Her family had been pressuring her to become the second wife of a wealthy businessman, whom she had never met, when she received a letter from the man who became her husband, the foreman of a road crew that had been working nearby:

> And the letter said, "Jessie, why are you hanging yourself up on this old man who already has a wife? (The verb *hangamapim*—to hang something up—can also mean to become attached or obligated to someone.) Have you met his wife? Have you thought about what your future will be like? Just wait a few days, and I will bring the same amount of bridewealth. If I don't, go ahead and marry him." [Did you know him?] No! I'd seen him working on the road, I knew his face, but we'd never spoken. I hadn't thought of him as a possible husband. I didn't know he was interested in me, and he only told me when he realized I was about to marry someone else.

Faced with a choice between two men she didn't know, one much older and married, and the other her age and unmarried, she "chose" the latter. Like Miriam and Helen, the emotional intimacy she had with her husband was accomplished in part through working as an economic team: he gave her some of his wages to invest in buying and selling betel nut:

> We made a lot of profit, and eventually I was able to invest in selling second-hand clothes and in raising chickens. We made a lot of profit from all our little businesses, and we were both very happy. We even made enough money so that we could buy a used car and a block of land. At the end of each day we would sit with our children and we would all count the money together. We would have a huge pile of coins and notes, and we would make smaller piles all worth K50 or K10 or K20. And we would talk together about what to do with it—this much for shopping, this much to save for the car, this much to buy more betel nut, this much for school fees. Like that.

Like Miriam, both Helen and Jessie were shocked when they learned their husbands had taken second wives. In the 2004 sample as a whole, the fathers of eighteen of the twenty-five women had two or more wives, so polygynous marriage was something almost all of them had grown up with, and arguably knew to expect. However, Miriam, Helen, Jessie, and a few others all had believed that their marriages were different from their mothers': they lived together with their husbands, they slept in the same room, they enjoyed sex with each other, they cooked and ate together, they planned, budgeted, and strategized together, and so on. In other words, they all felt they had achieved a degree of closeness, trust, and partnership with their husbands that was incompatible with polygyny. When they imagined the future and strategized with their husbands for how to accomplish specific goals, polygyny was not what they envisioned and was not part of the discussion.

These women felt betrayed in multiple ways when their husbands married second wives. Unsurprisingly, they felt a betrayal of the emotional intimacy and loyalty they thought they had established. They also felt a betrayal of their sense of being modern. Although everyone in Papua New Guinea knows that wealthy and powerful men, especially those from Highlands provinces, often take more than one wife, not all cultural groups in Papua New Guinea practice polygyny, and it is increasingly associated with being backwards, uneducated, and un-Christian. Thus, some women experienced a husband's taking a second wife as a humiliating temporal dislocation into a less civilized state. And since they were sometimes sent "back to the village," while the second wife remained with the husband, this temporal dislocation could become a very real spatial and economic dislocation. Finally, some women expressed a sense of having been betrayed in an additional temporal way: they felt that they and their husbands had been traveling along the same life path, and when a husband took another wife, it was as if he had abruptly left this shared path and reinvented himself as a newly young person with an array of life choices ahead of him. Alice, mother of three, and one of the few women who said she had married her *lawini* (her first true love) and continued to love her husband, had this to say about her husband's plan to marry another wife:

> We married when I was young and he was young. The same. We had children together and we have gotten older together. So why should he suddenly think he can turn young again and act like he is sixteen and take another wife. He can't look at me and decide that I am old but that he is suddenly young again! No! So I hit him. And I told him if he married a younger woman I would go have sex with a younger man. If he thinks he can be young again, so can I. But then he said he would cut my vagina if I did that, and I think he meant it. So I stopped saying that.

In sum, women's bitterness stems not only from feeling emotionally betrayed—particularly acute when one thought one's marriage was based on having "one name, one thought"—but also from the gendered unfairness of men's socially sanctioned ability to embark on a new life and to experience again the excitement of youthful desire and attachment. Being suddenly cast into the humiliating "savage slot" of being in a polygynous marriage only exacerbated this feeling of betrayal.

Marrying more than one wife is considered Huli men's right, and simply something most successful men do, unless they are devout Christians. Nevertheless, their sometimes underhanded ways of going about it indicate its increasingly contested nature. For example, Jessie's husband took another wife when she returned to Tari for a few months after her mother died. That he never came for the funeral and took advantage of her absence to surreptitiously marry a second wife seemed like the ultimate betrayal to her. Helen's husband lied to her and initially said his second wife was a cousin who needed a place to stay for a while. She was furious that she had welcomed this woman into her home, cooked for her, and had even given her some money, only to learn later that her husband had given bridewealth for her and was building her a house on a block of land that Helen had helped to purchase.

Men, unsurprisingly, view polygyny quite differently—the element of betrayal pales before its value as a strategic move, a source of prestige, and a display of powerful masculinity. Like the women, most of the men interviewed in 2004 had polygynous fathers, and although some resented a father's inability to pay the school fees of all of his children (for men this seemed to be the one significant and growing deterrent to polygyny), most spoke with pleasure of belonging to a large extended network of half-siblings. Many did not make much of a distinction between their own mother's children and the other wives' children, referring to all of them equally as brothers and sisters. Those whose fathers had three or more wives expressed pride at being the son of a man who was widely known to have many wives, children, pigs, and areas of land on a range of clan territories. Being able to marry more than one wife both demonstrated a man's wealth and might enable him to become even wealthier if his wives were good pig herders or were able to make a success of selling betel nut or second-hand clothes. Politicians were also more likely to court polygynous men with many adult children, since it was assumed that if the patriarch of a large, polygynous family directed every-one to vote for a particular candidate, they all would. Where monogamous mar-riage suggested a constricted sociality and was associated with an unmasculine Christian piety, polygynous marriage was associated with an admirable embrace of masculine desire for sex, social expansiveness, and political influence.

Wealthier men who had, or were angling for, leadership positions often mar-ried quite strategically so as to consolidate wealth or expand social connections. For example, Jethro, a young man I knew from my doctoral fieldwork in the 1990s (mentioned in chapter 1), had claims to a large number of the electrical pylons running from Hides to Porgera, which provided a handsome annual income. He made a point of marrying Daisy, whose older brother Monty had made money from buying and selling gold during the Mt. Kare gold rush (Clark 1993, Vail 1995, Biersack 1999, Wardlow 2001) and had invested it in trade stores and PMVs. Together the two men were able to expand their businesses into the Porgera area, and Jethro solidified his social and entrepreneurial connections there by taking a Porgeran wife who belonged to a landowning clan. Jethro's older sister, Theresa (see chapter 1), further expanded their social network there when she married a Porgeran policeman. Sadly, all the people in this story—Jethro and his two wives, Monty and his wife, and Theresa—became infected with HIV, and only Theresa was still alive in 2012, when I interviewed her.

These brother-sister pairs (Monty/Daisy, Jethro/Theresa) were two of the cases of siblings infected with HIV that made me suspect that HIV was significantly more prevalent in the Tari area than in Papua New Guinea as a whole. However, it is important to note that the HIV infection of these two sibling pairs can be seen as strongly socially determined: because polygyny is an important entrepre-neurial strategy for enhancing claims to land and recruiting partners for business ventures, an economic tie to a family can also be a sexual tie. Jethro, for example, had a sexual tie to Monty, both in the sense that he married Monty's sister, but also because, as business partners, they went out drinking together at the same hotel bars and joined the same sexual networks. Very likely, they slept with some of the same women. Moreover, business opportunities are most available in resource-extraction sites where, as discussed in chapter 1, landowners have preferential access to contracts for construction, catering, cleaning services, and other business opportunities, and can also exert control over which outside small businesses come into the area. Thus, an economic strategy (expanding one's PMV services) is also often a geographic strategy (expanding them into the Porgera area), which is also often a social strategy (drinking and womanizing with potential Porgeran business partners), as well as a marital strategy (taking a Porgeran woman as a second wife in order to gain permission for expansion of the PMV business). For entrepreneurial men, then, an economic strategy can easily become an array of HIV exposures for themselves and their wives.

MEN'S EXTRAMARITAL SEX

If polygyny is one source of conflict in marriage, as well as a source of HIV vulnerability, men's extramarital interactions are another (see also Lepani 2008). Twenty-two of the twenty-five women I interviewed in 2004 had been married to husbands who engaged in extramarital sex, though the number of other partners their husbands had likely varied tremendously. Ten of these women believed they had been infected with a sexually transmitted infection by their husband. (I say "believed" because I did not examine their clinic books for a diagnosis, and thus it is impossible to be sure that these were all STIs and not some other kind of vaginal infection.) And, as mentioned at the outset of this chapter, at least twenty-two of the thirty HIV-positive women I interviewed in 2012 and 2013 had been infected by their husbands.[3]

It is important to emphasize that little in precolonial Huli society promoted or condoned extramarital sex by either women or men. As discussed earlier, men were taught to protect their health and masculine vigor by living separately from women. Failure to abide by gender separation was said not only to compromise a man's health, but also the well-being of his male kin and allies, particularly if they were about to make war, and even to sap vitality from their land. Pre- or extramarital sex is considered a kind of theft from a woman's natal family or husband, and usually causes "trouble" (retaliatory violence, demands for compensation). And because of the spousal corporeal porosity discussed earlier, wives and children are said to experience malaise, weakness, and sometimes worse when husbands "jump over them" (*kalapim ol;* that is, stray sexually). Indeed, men are often quite anxious about how their extramarital forays might negatively impact or be "felt" by their wives and children, and some make a point of drinking and washing in the purest mountain water they can find before coming home, hoping that this will act as a kind of cleansing prophylaxis against any damage to the household that might result from their liaisons. In short, when seeking to explain why a high proportion of married men might have extramarital sex, precolonial philosophies and practices regarding sex provide no answers; if anything, they worked to discourage, prevent, and punish extramarital sex.

Of the many changes instigated by the colonial and postcolonial periods, most important in fostering extramarital sex has been male labor migration, originating with the Highlands Labor Scheme, implemented in 1950 to help Australian colonial plantations recover from the devastation of World War II by bringing men from the densely populated inland, mountainous areas down to the coast for short periods of labor (Ward 1990). The economic trajectory of the Southern Highlands region, including the Tari area, was profoundly shaped by this scheme. The initial areas of labor recruitment—the Eastern and later Western Highlands regions—were also the areas where families were encouraged to establish their own coffee gardens in order to supplement the output of Australian-owned plantations. By the early 1960s, indigenous smallholder coffee production had overtaken the colonists' plantation production, and by the mid 1960s it had exceeded Australia's export quota (Stewart 1992, Good 1986, West 2012). Consequently, in order to limit coffee production and ensure the availability of labor for coastal plantations, the colonial administration extended its labor recruitment to more remote highlands areas, such as Southern Highlands Province, and never developed these areas as coffee producers (Strathern 1982, Connell 2005). From the mid 1960s until 1974, when the scheme ended, most of the workers came from Southern Highlands Province (Ward 1990, Harris 1972, Fitzpatrick 1980). High levels of male out-migration from the area continued even after this period: migration data from 1982, for example, show that in some areas around Tari, approximately 45 percent of men between the ages of 20 and 39 were absent from their home communities (Lehmann 2002, Lehmann et al. 1997).

This history—of being far from Highlands centers of economic power, of never developing the coffee economies that Eastern Highlands Province and Western Highlands Province did, and, especially, of spending often long periods away from home in search of economic opportunity—has shaped Huli discourses about themselves as a people, as well as notions of masculinity. For example, throughout the 2000s, I often heard Huli claim that they were "the slaves of the nation" because of their past history of helping other provinces to develop (while their own province languished) through their labor for plantations, infrastructure projects, mines, and so on. And, migration in search of economic opportunity is now an expected part of masculine experience for Huli men. Of the fifty-four men my male field assistants interviewed in 2004, thirty-one (57 percent) had spent six months or more working in another area of Papua New Guinea, typically in mines, on tea or copra plantations, or as store clerks or security guards in urban centers. Many described how migrant male friendships were forged and maintained through drinking, buying sex, joking about sexual liaisons, and sharing information about sexual partners. A number of them complained about the peer pressure to engage in these activities, and lamented the guilt they felt about spending money on personal pleasures instead of sending money home (Wardlow 2009, Hirsch et al. 2010).

But if being far from home and in the company of other male migrants often initiates what might be called a man's extramarital sexual debut, this does not mean that extramarital liaisons are confined to places away from home. And because of the disappearance of other ways for women to make money in and around Tari, it was easy to find sex for sale there by the 2000s, as discussed in chapter 2.

WIVES REACT: VIOLENCE AND *BEKIM BEK*

Gender inequality among the Huli allows men great freedom of mobility and little obligation to account for their time spent away from home, privileges generally denied to wives. Thus, as one AIDS educator announced to her all-female audience when trying to counter their religious objections to her speaking publicly about condoms: "What? You think you can carry your husband's cock around in your string bag? Men go where they want and do what they want, and they take their cocks with them." Unable to prevent a husband's extramarital forays, many wives have to decide how to respond to their knowledge about them. In some cases, women respond by ignoring their increasing suspicions or by pretending they don't know, until circumstances, such as experiencing symptoms of a sexually transmitted infection, provide them with a morally irreproachable rationale (protecting their fertility) for broaching the subject.

Angry or even violent confrontation was at least as common a response to male infidelity. Although male privilege explicitly sanctions many freedoms denied to women, it does not include *anguatole* or *kelapim* (Huli and Tok Pisin, respectively, for jumping or stepping over someone, euphemisms for extramarital sex), and Christian missionization has reinforced the idea that extramarital sex is immoral. Moreover, unlike in other cultural contexts where a husband's extramarital sorties are often attributed to his wife's supposed failings, and are thus a source of shame to her (Hirsch et al. 2010), Huli men's affairs are generally attributed to their own desires and weaknesses. Thus, many Huli women show no compunction about making a spectacle of a husband's dalliances by demanding compensation in village court or by physically attacking him and his partner in public. Indeed, many of the women I interviewed seemed to fear losing face if they *didn't* expose a husband's affair and attempt to punish him for it. Eleven of the twenty-two women I interviewed in 2004 who said they knew their husbands had engaged in extramarital sex spoke of responding violently.

Miriam, whose story began this chapter, physically attacked her second husband (the one she had moved in with after meeting him at a *dawe anda*) when she learned he continued to have sex with other women:

[Has there been a time when your husband made you very angry?] Yes. He had sex at a *dawe anda*. I told him not to go, but he went anyway and had sex with a woman I know. And then they continued having sex for three months. He would sleep at our house, but go have sex with her during the day. And I lost weight, and I was tired all the time. I just wanted to sleep. I was very weak. And finally I confronted him. I said, "I think you must be having sex with another woman." Because some women told me that if your husband is having sex with other women, you will feel tired and weak. So I asked him, and he denied it. But one day I followed him, and I saw him ask this woman for money so that he could play cards. A man only asks his wife or sister for money, so I picked up a stick, ran up to him, and whipped him in the face and head. I was really angry with him then.

Maria, a woman who looked to be in her late thirties, also responded violently when she was confronted with her husband's infidelity, though her marriage had long been conflict-ridden. She described herself as having grown up in a very traditional family. Her father had five wives (her mother was the second wife), and he lived in his own house:

He was a man who followed custom. He rarely visited his wives, and when his wives gave birth, he never came to look at the baby. And his house wasn't nearby—it was very far away from our house. We never saw him.

When she was in grade one, her father informed her that she would be marrying an acquaintance of his:

I didn't know him. My father knew him. My father just came and announced that I had to go marry this older man. . . . I was very young. Only grade one. I didn't have breasts yet. I hadn't started menstruating. I was married to my husband for two years before I got my period. (Huli children often don't start grade one until age ten, and in the past, when Maria would have been in school, the starting age was often older.)

In fact, Maria didn't meet her husband until two years after marrying him because he was living in Port Moresby, and his family gave bridewealth to hers in his absence:

When he came back from Port Moresby I wanted us to have separate rooms. I was very young, and he was much older, but he said no, and he insisted on having sex. He found it very difficult to get inside me. I bled, but he couldn't get it all the way in. To make it more slippery, he tried lathering his penis with soap, but that was very painful and it didn't work. Then he lathered his penis with cooking oil, and that worked. And I got pregnant very quickly, which made him angry because he wanted to keep having sex with me, and I said no. This is our custom, and I was afraid that if we kept having sex it would damage me or the baby. So I ran home and stayed with my parents. But he sent the police to fetch me back.

Throughout their marriage they argued and sometimes physically fought about sex: she showed me small scars on her head, legs, and arms where he had cut her with a knife for refusing sex, and she had one very long, thick scar on her arm from when he had tried to cut her with a knife and she had thrown up her arm in defense:

> But I hit him too. I stabbed him too. Once I stabbed him in public, in front of Bromley's (Tari's largest store through the 1990s until 2002, when it was looted and then closed; see chapter 2). I was retaliating because he had almost cut my arm off. He had to go to the hospital for stitches. I used to be a bad woman (*meri nogut,* which literally means a bad woman, but is usually used to mean a fierce, unforgiving woman): if he cut me, I would cut him back. If he poked me with a knife, I poked him back. I only thought about getting revenge. But it was all because of sex. He wanted sex all the time.

Although she resisted what she experienced as his excessive demands for sex, Maria was nevertheless enraged when she came upon her husband having sex with another woman one night:

> He had sold a pig and had money to spend. So he went to a *dawe anda* near our house and found a woman there. And I discovered them. . . . I thought I heard our pig squealing, and I grabbed a large bush knife. I thought someone was stealing our pig. So I ran with a big bush knife, and I came upon the two of them bare naked and fucking [You saw them naked?] Yes, I saw their asses and their other sexual parts. I was so embarrassed and angry. I yelled, "What are you doing? You're fucking this woman?" And my husband yelled, "You always say you don't want to have sex, so yes, I found someone else to fuck." And I tried to cut the woman with the bush knife, but he grabbed me and held my arms to my sides. And I yelled at him, "Don't touch me. You just had sex. Get away from me. Don't touch my skin." And he wrestled the knife away from me and threw it aside. So I grabbed the woman's clothes and her bag and threw them into the stream nearby. She was naked and had no clothes.
>
>   And then I started yelling as loud as I could. And a bunch of men came running, and they saw her standing there naked, and then they held her legs and arms and took her away and fucked her. [Are you saying they took her away and raped her? (I'd been chuckling at her throwing the woman's clothes into a stream, but you can hear the shock enter my voice.)] Yes, they raped her. There were lots of men and just her, and she was naked. [Why did they do that?] Because I told them to. When I was yelling for them to come, I said, "There's a woman in my pig house. You all take her and fuck her. She's looking for men." My husband didn't go with them. He came back to my house, but I told him to go away. I told him he fucked around with passenger women, and I didn't care if killed a pig for me (that is, gave her compensation for "jumping over" her). I told him he was a gonorrhea man and I didn't want to see him.

That women expose other women to men's sexual violence is rare, but does happen. Recall from chapter 1, for example, that Kelapi's uncle's wife conspired with their Porgeran landowner patron to abduct her and take her as his wife. Women may do this for pragmatic reasons, as in the case of Kelapi's aunt, who wanted to maintain good relations with their landowner patron. Or they may, like Maria, want to punish women they feel have humiliated them. Also important in Maria's case, I think, is the chronic conflict and violence that she had experienced in her marriage, starting with what amounted to marital rape at a very young age, which led her, according to her own account, to become more angry and violent herself. To be clear, Maria did not actually witness the woman being raped by the men she had summoned with her shouting, and Huli women's narratives about violent confrontation are often characterized by a triumphalist tone (Wardlow 2006a) in which a female narrator's successes are amplified and her nemesis's iniquitous nature, and consequent downfall, are exaggerated. In such narratives, the humiliation of the female nemesis, often through her public nudity (Wardlow 2006a: 91), is emphasized. Nevertheless, regardless of how Maria might have embroidered this narrative, her tacit assertion is that sexual violence is a morally acceptable or even appropriate retribution against a husband's illegitimate sexual partner, particularly if the woman attends *dawe anda* or is a passenger woman. Maria's attitude indicates her fury about her husband's bringing a sexual partner onto their territory, an act that both polluted the land and demonstrated his disregard for her. This narrative also indicates the way that women who are categorized as sexually transgressive can precipitously be thrust into an abject status that makes them be seen as deserving recipients of punitive sexual violence. In other words, despite an apparent increase in tolerance for women who engage in transactional sex in Tari (see chapter 2), in fact it takes very little to expel such women from a moral space of safety (see also Kelly-Hanku et al. 2016).

Women also sometimes respond violently to a husband's decision to marry an additional wife. Helen, whose husband had found her a job as a hotel maid, said this, for example, about discovering that her husband's "cousin" was actually his second wife:

> There were two incidents when I cut that woman with a knife, and three times that I cut him with a knife. Once he had to go to the hospital and get eight stitches, and another time he had to get four stitches. Finally I said, "I might end up killing you, and then I would be causing a lot of trouble for my kin (meaning they would have to pay compensation for her murdering him). So tell the business to transfer you to some other hotel. We shouldn't live in the same place—I might end up dead, or you might end up dead, or she might end up dead. And then we are causing trouble for our kin."

While women often represent their physical aggression towards a husband and/or his extramarital partner as primarily an expression of uncontrollable rage, it does, in fact, have a purpose: it is intended to sever the extramarital relationship and drive the other woman away. Recall that when her husband's first wife attacked Theresa (see chapter 1), who was married to a policeman in Porgera, she responded with escalated aggression and compelled the other woman to leave.

Responding with *bekim bek*—revenge sex—was not quite as common as women's violent reactions to men's philandering. Seven of those in my 2004 sample of twenty-five married women responded to their husbands' infidelity—or, as in Miriam's case, his decision to take a second wife—with *bekim bek*. Tani, for example, had heard rumors that her husband was sleeping with her cousin, and

> I wanted to see for myself. So one day when I heard they were at it again I went and looked. Our house was a *haus kapa* (literally, house copper; that is, a modern house with a metal roof), and it had a window, so I could look inside (most "bush houses"—that is, houses built with the wood of local trees and grass—do not have windows). And there they were, drinking Gold Cup (whiskey) and listening to the radio. . . . So I left and went to stay with my kin, and I kept thinking and thinking, "How can I get the bridewealth returned? How can I get the bridewealth returned?" (In other words, she wondered how she might be able to divorce her husband, which would require the return of at least some of the bridewealth he had given for her.) And I realized it would be impossible. Because if your family chooses your husband and it goes badly, then they might return the bridewealth. But if you choose your own husband, like I did, then they won't. They will say, "You wanted him. We didn't choose him, you did. So stay with him." So I thought, "Okay, he wants to fuck my cousin, I'll go fuck his cousin. I will retaliate (*Bai mi bekim bek*)." And there was this man from T—, a really fat man. He was one of my in-laws, but he'd asked me to marry him when I was younger. I had refused because he already had a wife. But I went and found him, and he greeted me politely, but I just said it to him directly: "Your cousin is fucking my cousin. What do you think?" And he said, "Let's go." So I went and stayed with him for two weeks and had sex with him.

Since divorce seemed out of reach, Tani was aiming for exact adulterous equivalence: a cousin for a cousin. Anthropologists have often written about the Melanesian ethic and logic of reciprocity and equivalence, typically when analyzing gift exchange between individuals and groups. How this ethic can also inform interpersonal, and even sexual, relations has been less explored, however. Often women describe themselves as aiming for an *affective equivalence:* that is, they want to cause the same kind and degree of emotional pain that they themselves have experienced. In this case, Tani wanted to injure and insult her husband in the exact proportion that he had hurt her; moreover, she anticipated that when the inevitable fight about her behavior erupted, she would be able to assert this equivalence, and thus argue that she and her husband were even in terms of having wronged each other. She wanted to humiliate him by rubbing this adulterous equivalence in his face, but also wanted to limit the physically violent retaliation from him that she felt would be merited if she had gone beyond this equivalence and wronged him to a greater degree than he had wronged her.

It is also important to note that Tani, while aiming for equivalence, also chose her extramarital sexual partner safely in the sense of opting for someone familiar: an in-law who was also a former suitor. In contrast, most of the other women

who resorted to *bekim bek* chose partners unknown to them, the first ma
come along, as it were—or at least this is what they told me. Acting impulsi
and showing little deliberation (at least in recounting it, and perhaps in their
actual behavior) was a way of demonstrating their extreme rage and its uncontrollable nature.

CONCLUSION

In the public health literature about HIV, polygyny is often treated as a risk factor: it is referred to as "marital concurrency," which is conceptualized as a form of
"sexual concurrency"—that is, having more than one sexual partner at the same
time (as opposed to having serial sexual partners one after the other), a mode of
sexual partnering that is thought by many epidemiologists to pose greater HIV
risk (Halperin and Epstein 2004, Mah and Halperin 2010). Polygyny is assumed
to be hazardous because if one of the spouses contracts HIV, it may spread to the
others: a husband can infect not just one wife, but two or more. This framework
assumes a particular model of polygyny in which a husband continues to have sex
with his existing wife or wives after taking a new one. While this is often true, there
are, in fact, a variety of ways in which polygyny unfolds among the Huli, particularly as it has become more controversial and contested.[4] In some cases, when a
man takes a second wife, the first wife will refuse to continue having sex with him,
citing fear of disease, anger about the loss of resources for herself and her children,
or simply, "I've given you children, now it's her turn."

It is clear from my interviews that (1) marital concurrency isn't necessarily
sexual concurrency and, in fact, may sometimes look a lot more like serial sexual
partnering, and (2) polygyny, at least among the Huli, can take such a wide range
of lived forms that it cannot be considered a stable and coherent independent variable or risk factor. Also problematic is that the public health framework of "marital
concurrency" assumes a kind of temporal stasis, in which polygyny is treated as
a person's stable trait. A more dynamic approach (that is, a more ethnographic
approach) would examine how all the spouses in a marriage enact and respond
to polygyny. It could very well be that polygyny poses increased HIV risk, but not
necessarily because the infection of one spouse leads to the infection of all. Rather,
a woman's anger about a new wife might drive her to *bekim bek* with multiple
partners, exposing her to HIV. Alternatively, or additionally, abandoned by her
husband as his affections turn towards his new wife, she might engage in transactional sex in order to provide for herself and her children.

In addition to the dramatic economic and political upheavals discussed in
chapters 1 and 2, Huli have also experienced a great deal of upheaval in the marital
domain. A generation ago, most married couples lived in separate houses and saw
little of each other, but now most live together in one house—an enormous change,
not only in the structure and composition of households, but also in spouses'

affective lives. Many Huli find this challenging—perhaps especially the current generation of men, who have been raised to be wary about excessive bodily contact with women, feel trepidation about "knowing each other too well," and are often unprepared for managing the challenges of this kind of marriage.

These challenges are exacerbated by men's and women's differing desires and aspirations for marriage. While both men and women want to be able to choose their own spouses, women typically have greater aspirations that their marriages will be companionate—that is, emotionally fulfilling and characterized by a real partnership of shared goals, joint decision-making, and communication about sex and reproduction. They hope that this kind of partnership precludes polygyny. Men, while often enjoying the pleasures and benefits of a shared house and a wife's companionship, are reluctant to relinquish household authority, absolute freedom of movement, the pleasures of extramarital relations, and the rewards of polygyny, which include prestige and the potential for creating a large, economically power-ful, and politically influential family. Women like Miriam, Helen, and Jessie hope, and sometimes allow themselves to assume, that what they experience as a foun-dation of intimacy, trust, and good communication will protect them from polyg-yny. However, women like these may be those most at risk of finding themselves in a polygynous marriage: the upward mobility and economic success they have achieved as economic partners with their husbands contribute to their feelings of joyous connection, but this very success enables their husbands to take additional wives. In point of fact, of the twenty-five married women I interviewed in 2004, eighteen of their first marriages were either initially or eventually polygynous, by which I mean that they either married as second wives or they were first wives whose husbands eventually took one or more additional wives.

In light of the violent conflict that often erupts over clashing marital expecta-tions, it is not surprising that organizations like Population Services International have developed marital training workshops to help couples try to understand each other's perspectives and communicate in ways that reduce the likelihood of physi-cal aggression. It is tempting to analyze such workshops as biopolitical interven-tions aimed at producing compliant, affectively self-regulating marital subjects. The workshop handbook does, after all, employ exercises that encourage partici-pants to be more self-reflective about their emotions and gives them lots of prac-tice in translating explosive negative feelings into less volatile verbal formulations. In short, seeing these workshops through a Foucauldian lens would be analyti-cally fruitful. Nevertheless, given the anger and desolation expressed by many men and women about their marriages in the 2004 interviews, it would seem a good idea to equip couples with skills that might help them strive for the companionate marriages to which many aspire. In essence, such workshops "de-naturalize" com-panionate marriage by acknowledging that specific, difficult skills are required to make it work, and that many couples the world over find it challenging.

The idea, however, that such workshops might have a significant impact on HIV vulnerability seems highly optimistic. As discussed in this chapter and the previous two, there are many factors that shape men's and women's sexual behavior, including the long history of Huli men's migration out of Tari to find work and the economic downturn that drove many women to engage in transactional sex. Workshops like the one offered by PSI presume a couple in which both partners are present and co-habiting—not estranged by polygyny or migrant labor—and thus do not directly confront the structural factors that have created HIV vulnerability.

4

Teaching Gender to Prevent AIDS

I can't feed my baby beard hair to make her grow a beard and become a man. She is a girl. This won't change. That is sex. Jenda *is what you learn in life that gives you power. For example, you learn to be a pilot or you learn to be a nurse.* Jenda *is important because you can change it. If you are sinful, you can become a religious man. If you are a woman who plays cards and gambles, you can change and become a woman who plants sweet potatoes.* Jenda *is the things you can change.*

—ANNA, AN AIDS EDUCATOR

During a week-long AIDS Awareness workshop at a health center not far from Tari, this was one of the ways the instructor explained the difference between sex and gender to the participants. As noted in chapter 3, AIDS education in the Tari area in the early 2010s was animated by a "will to improve" (Li 2007) gender relations, and especially marital relations. "Improvement" entailed both promoting gender equality and equipping married couples with communication and other skills for making marital relations more harmonious. Educating people about the difference between sex (as biologically based) and gender (as culturally constructed) seemed to be an important step in this work of improvement.

I was initially flummoxed by this goal of teaching workshop participants, many of whom had very little formal education and were not fluent in English, about the difference between sex and gender, terms that have no equivalent in Huli or Tok Pisin. What did this have to do with preventing HIV transmission?

The logic behind this pedagogical aim had two parts. The first is that gender inequality drives the global HIV pandemic and makes women and girls disproportionately vulnerable to infection. Factors such as women's early marriage, their lower educational and employment levels, their economic dependency and lesser control over land and other assets, and their inability to control when and how sex takes place all contribute to their greater vulnerability, as do masculine prestige structures that reward men for acquiring many sexual partners (Mannell 2010, Mukherjee and Das 2011, Hirsch et al. 2010). In Papua New Guinea, all these factors, as well as very high rates of sexual and domestic violence (Borrey 2000, Lepani 2008, MSF 2010, Jolly et al. 2012, Biersack et al. 2016), have spurred AIDS prevention approaches that focus on confronting and dismantling gender inequality (Seeley and Butcher 2006, Hammar 2010). Second, confronting and dismantling gender inequality is thought to require (among many other things) conveying the cultural constructedness of gender roles and making visible the part that societies play in valuing, and granting power to, the male gender over the female gender. Thus, to combat women's HIV vulnerability, one must understand that this vulnerability is created, in part, by gendered roles and values, which, since they are not determined by biological sex, can (and should) be changed.

During this AIDS education workshop, the concept of gender was presented, erased, and transformed over the course of the week. In this chapter I juxtapose how gender was supposed to be taught, according to the workshop handbook, with how it was presented and explained by Anna, the AIDS educator, demonstrating the important role that these educators play in knowledge transmission, as well as the ways in which they can transform the information they convey (Wardlow 2012). *Jenda*—the neologism I use, following Anna's pronunciation, in order to distinguish it from the English term "gender"—can, like gender, be contrasted with sex, but is only loosely tied to it, and is more about acquiring empowering skills (e.g., becoming a nurse) or about moral work on the self (e.g., giving up gambling) than about gendered relations of power or cultural elaborations of the sexed body. A central critique articulated by Anna was that the handbook's discussions of gender, gender inequality, and gender-based violence represented men and women as antagonistically opposed, rather than as complementarily joined or interdependent, which she found inaccurate and unhelpful, and which motivated her efforts to redefine the concept of gender. However, despite her efforts to render gender into a conceptual tool for human betterment (that is, *jenda*), anger about gender inequality sporadically erupted during the workshop, almost causing it to fall apart.

The ideas about gender presented in the workshop handbook—that sex is biological and gender is social; that gendered tasks are variable around the world, suggesting gender's plastic and arbitrary nature; but that male dominance and female subordination are nevertheless pervasive—are all directly inspired by feminist anthropological research. And despite the problematization of the sex/gender binary by anthropological and other scholarly work, gender nevertheless has canonical status as an emancipatory and empowering concept, particularly when opposed to the constriction and determinism associated with its dyadic partner, biological sex. That an AIDS educator in Papua New Guinea did not find the idea of gender to be emancipatory or empowering challenges hard-won intellectual battles, and suggests the need to examine the kind of conceptual work we assume that the sex/gender binary does and why it might not accomplish this same work in other contexts.

A BRIEF HISTORY OF HIV/AIDS EDUCATION IN TARI

As discussed in chapter 2, Tari, and much of Southern Highlands Province, was going through a tumultuous and sometimes violent socioeconomic decline in the early 2000s. Crime had increased significantly, and almost everyone I knew had stories to tell of being held up by armed gangs or pick-pocketed in the main market. Many NGOs declared Tari a "no-go zone," refusing to send their employees there. In this context, I felt that I could not ethically carry out research without giving something substantial in return. I also hoped that visibly providing a service might make local gangs decide to leave me alone.[1] So, it was for both self-protective and ethical reasons that I began doing AIDS education in the Tari area in 2004. In a bid to keep electrical power running to its gold mine after a year of ongoing sabotage, Porgera Joint Venture (PJV) had established a small Community Relations office in Tari, employing local men as liaisons to the areas where power pylons were located. Since the local hospital, which had suffered great reductions in its staff, could not spare any resources for my efforts, I eventually proposed that this PJV office assist me. It is perhaps no surprise that it was happy to support my attempts at AIDS education: the two expatriate managers (who worked in rotation, each with approximately two weeks on and two weeks off) were trying to project a benevolent image for PJV, while their Huli staff shared my concern that people in the Tari area were highly vulnerable to HIV.

Choosing to collaborate with a mining company to provide health education might appear questionable (cf. Welker 2016), so I provide some context here. First, my AIDS education effort was never officially supported by PJV: it had no dedicated funding or staff; rather, the expatriate managers provided, when they could spare them, a vehicle, one or more community liaison officers, and a driver. In fact, they didn't initially document the AIDS awareness activities in their reports for fear that their supervisors in Porgera would quash an ad hoc project that had not been formally initiated and approved from above. At that time there was little direct oversight of PJV's small office in Tari, affording the expatriate managers a great deal of autonomy, and they both strongly favored a benevolent developmentalist approach to "asset protection" (that is, protecting the power pylons from sabotage), rather than punitive policing measures. Thus, they often used their discretionary funds to support small local projects, and they perceived AIDS education as an important addition to the services they were providing.

I was also strongly encouraged by my female friends, especially local women's group leaders and the women who ran my guesthouse, to forge ties with this office because, with many government offices and private businesses closed or abandoned, it was the primary source of technical and other resources in Tari. These women fully recognized that it was my white status that enabled my easy entrance through the compound's high, guarded gates—when they themselves might have had to wait in line for hours—and they wanted to exploit that status as best they could. Every time I went to the PJV office to organize an AIDS awareness presentation, they armed me with requests for funds, equipment, and technical services (such as fixing generators or leaky water tanks), many of which I was able to help them secure. Moreover, the Huli employees at the office were very concerned about their communities' vulnerability to HIV and lack of information about AIDS, and they continually urged me to increase the number of presentations we were doing. On balance I felt that using my white privilege to obtain assets, influence, and services needed by local women's groups and to provide basic information about AIDS outweighed the problematic possibility that my collaboration with PJV might help burnish its image, precisely at a time when it was trying to build peaceable community relations.

When my 2004 fieldwork was nearing completion, and in the interests of making the work of AIDS education sustainable, the expatriate managers granted my request to send one of my field assistants and some of their staff to Port Moresby for official training and accreditation from the PNG National AIDS Council. A number of these individuals proved to be dedicated, gifted, and cherished AIDS educators who continued to improve their knowledge and skills through participation in numerous HIV/AIDS training programs, and they were later employed by a wide range of NGOs, churches, and businesses, eventually making Hela a place where AIDS education was relatively widespread.

AIDS EDUCATION: DANGEROUS KNOWLEDGE AND THE ANTHROPOLOGY OF IGNORANCE

When I began new fieldwork in Tari in 2010, the socioeconomic landscape had changed dramatically. PJV still maintained an office in Tari, but, with the construction phase of ExxonMobil's liquid natural gas project at its height, and with government funds pouring in for the new Hela Province, PJV's influence was much diminished in Tari. By then a number of NGOs were engaged in AIDS awareness, as were some churches, and Oil Search (one of the PNG LNG joint venture partners) also employed staff to carry out AIDS education. For the sake of protecting the identity of the AIDS educator who conducted the workshop I discuss in this chapter, I do not identify the organization to which she belonged. This is somewhat problematic since the reader might wonder whether the employing organization—corporate entity, NGO, or religious institution—could exert significant influence over the content presented. And while this is a reasonable question, in fact all the AIDS educators I met or observed received standardized training and certification from the PNG National AIDS Council, and when carrying out AIDS education, they were expected to follow the manual with which they were equipped. There was a specific set of topics that they were expected to cover in a particular way, and they were trained in specific exercises, examples, and metaphors for illustrating various points. In other words, much of what they were supposed to do was literally scripted. Thus, the employing agency exerted less influence over workshop content than one might think. That said, one of my aims is to show how AIDS educators do exert translational agency in explicating the content of the AIDS Council manual in their own way, often based on their own reservations about the material.

Anna did, for the most part, follow the handbook quite closely. It is instructive, then, to attend to just where and why she departed from it, which was regarding gender. Arguably, international donor organizations and the Papua New Guinea National AIDS Council might identify gender-related information as what Papua New Guineans—and especially Huli—perhaps need most of all. However, these were the points where Anna most disagreed with the script she was supposed to follow.

In this specific workshop there were twenty participants, ten men and ten women. All of them were or had been married. Two-thirds of them were Huli speakers, and the rest were from other areas of Papua New Guinea and had either married into the area or had been assigned there (e.g., as church pastors). Approximately two-thirds of them were not functionally literate in English, either because they had never attended school or because they had attended long ago and had not since used their knowledge of English. Most of them had been invited because they were leaders in the community (pastors, clan leaders, women's group leaders). The hope was that as leaders they would act as "agents of change," disseminating what they learned to their respective constituencies.

In fact, at the beginning of the workshop the participants were anxious and unsure about whether they wanted to learn about HIV at all. While they were proud to have been chosen, they were also wary about how participation might damage their reputations or confront them with information about sex that they feared could be morally corrupting and that they felt shouldn't be shared widely. The AIDS education workshop—seemingly a straightforward site in which basic biomedical and public health knowledge is conveyed—in this instance turned out to be a complex epistemological and ethical space, where the instructor and participants carefully navigated between the Scylla and Charybdis of knowledge and ignorance. The literature in the "anthropology of ignorance" proves fruitful for analyzing this complex space and how the participants positioned themselves within it. For one thing, this literature suggests that relations of inequality are sustained and reproduced through the discursive production of some people as lacking necessary knowledge. For example, the global AIDS assemblage (Nguyen 2008) operates in part by imagining and discursively producing particular places as urgently in need of absent knowledge about sexual transmission, viruses, immune systems, condoms, and health-promoting gender relations. And the dissemination of biomedical health knowledge is therefore assumed to be an inherently valuable endeavor with health- and life-saving potential.

In contrast, anthropologists have observed that not-knowing can be experienced and valued as socially and morally protective. Ilana Gershon and Dhooleka Sarhadi Raj (2000: 3) suggest that it is ethnographically productive to investigate when and why "people actively construct, claim, and maintain ignorance for themselves." Casey High argues, for example, that among the Amazonian Waorani, knowing about shamanism can position the knower as a potential predator in relation to other living beings; "rejecting that knowledge, actively 'unknowing' it is therefore a way of avoiding the predator's perspective and maintaining peaceful relationships with their peers" (Mair, Kelly, and High 2012: 18; High 2012). Moreover, while ignorance or not-knowing is typically presumed to be a kind of empty epistemological space, devoid of content, Mair et al. suggest that it may, in fact, be substantively very meaningful: "There is an *ideology*, an *ethics*, and a *phenomenology* of ignorance," they say (Mair, Kelly, and High 2012: 5; emphasis added). This describes well how Huli understand the customary practice of rigorously not-knowing about sex prior to marriage. The *ideology* of this not-knowing might be summarized as: sex is physically damaging to young men because it saps them of their vitality and causes premature aging, and it is morally damaging to young women because "opening them up" unleashes their desires for sexual pleasure. Strict ignorance about sex is the only way to prevent these dangers, and marriage the safest way to encompass and control them. The *ethics* of premarital not-knowing about sex is that community cooperation in sustaining ignorance prevents social harm because premarital sex can embroil young people's families in bitter disputes. The *phenomenology* of sexual ignorance is the feeling of purity, vitality, and well-being while in the state of not-knowing, and, conversely, the sensation of alarm, violation, or deep embarrassment when one is inappropriately exposed to sexual knowledge. Thus, for example, the one young unmarried man mistakenly invited to participate in this particular AIDS workshop stood up and fled after he skimmed the handbook, which had line drawings of reproductive parts and condoms.

The other participants also expressed concerns about the handbook and seemed to be struggling with two competing ethical orientations towards the workshop. Far from being a meta activity a step or more removed from sex, they suggested, the workshop might itself be a sexual activity, in that it entailed looking at drawings of sexual organs and hearing information about sex, both of which could be sexually arousing. From this perspective, agreeing to be a participant was prurient, something only someone with an unhealthy sexual appetite (a *tanga bubu* in Huli, or "sex maniac," as some of the participants said) would do. Where researchers, health educators, and science more generally would prefer to see a behavior or practice (e.g., sex) as ontologically distinct from the meta-discourse about it (e.g., "AIDS awareness"), target audiences do not automatically accept that the behavior and the discourse are separate and qualitatively different, and they do not necessarily experience the latter as non-sexual. Janna Flora, trying to investigate motivations for suicide in a circumpolar population in Greenland, similarly encountered a reluctance to discuss the topic, because "talking about suicide, sometimes even in general terms, is perceived as dangerous in that it can provoke thoughts of suicide; thoughts that in turn can become directed toward an intended suicide" (Flora 2012: 148). In other words, talk, even when demarcated as a specific meta-discursive genre (e.g., interview, educational presentation) characterized by its own technical lexicon and interactional style, can never truly have a relationship external to the activity it describes or asks about, because talk is always intimately tied to affect, impulse, and desire. There is always the possibility that talk of a forbidden or taboo act might lure the ever-desiring mind closer to the doing of the act.

The other competing moral orientation towards the workshop was that since AIDS was a new and fatal, yet preventable, disease, learning about it was the enlightened, ethical, and necessary thing for leaders to do if they wanted to help their communities. Anna actively encouraged this latter orientation by using a range of framing and participatory strategies to represent workshop participation as the right moral choice. For example, she reminded the participants daily that they were there because, "as good Christians, everyone here is dedicated to saving the lives of people in the community and saving Huli culture." This phrase was intended to accomplish a few things. First, it framed learning about AIDS as religious practice, rather than irreligious prurient desire. Second, it represented the stakes as not only individual lives, but also Huli culture: AIDS could take such a devastating toll on households and communities, Anna suggested, that Huli culture itself would start to disintegrate. She thereby simultaneously appealed to the participants' ethno-nationalist sentiments—sentiments that were strong at the time, because of the creation of the new Hela Province—and assuaged some of their fears. Anna also began and ended each day by calling on one of the male pastors to give a short sermon and by asking one of the women to lead the group in prayer. And she made a point of interpellating the participants almost as children, and cultivating in them a kind of innocence, by starting each session with clapping games or children's songs. In short, acknowledging that the workshop content was morally complicated, she sought to create the space of the workshop, and the participants in it, as virtuous.

TEACHING GENDER

Much of Stacy Pigg's description of AIDS education workshops in Nepal (2001, 2005) also applies to this workshop, suggesting that such workshops follow much the same procedure everywhere. Anna explained the acronyms HIV and AIDS; the immune system and how HIV disables it; AIDS-related symptoms and disease progression; true and untrue modes of HIV transmission (e.g., sexual transmission versus sharing utensils); various means of prevention, including abstinence, fidelity to one partner, and condom use; and the basic workings of the male and female reproductive systems. These topics were organized into sessions, with two or three sessions covered each day. All of the above topics were explained much as the handbook laid out the information.

Where Anna deviated from the script of the handbook was in her explanation of the concept of gender. She understood that gender referred to the culturally variable roles and behaviors that were expected of men and women, but she disagreed with some of the handbook's assertions and implications. She declared, for example, that some of the behaviors or capacities described by the handbook as culturally constructed were, in fact, determined by sex. She also skipped most of the handbook's sections on gender inequality and gender-based violence, feeling that the representation of these topics was reductive, overly inflammatory, and unproductive in the goal of improving marital relations. Finally, she felt that the concept of gender, indicating as it did a large degree of behavioral plasticity, was better deployed to encourage participants to improve themselves morally. In short, when it came to the topics about gender, and only the topics about gender, she took a highly agentive, or even activist, stance in her role as instructor and translator (cf. Tymoczko 2010, Venuti 2008).

Sex or Gender?

One of the learning objectives in the handbook is for participants to understand the difference between sex and gender, with sex defined as "the biological attributes of being either male or female . . . it is fixed and cannot be changed," and gender defined as "socially constructed. It is made up of learned attributes and behaviours. You are not born with your gender. It is your learned identity. . . .It can be changed" (PNG NAC 2007, 30). The ultimate goal is to show that biologically essentialist notions of men and women often limit women's autonomy, restrict their opportunities, and naturalize expectations of female obedience to male authority, thereby exacerbating women's vulnerability to HIV. Gender as social construction, in contrast, is intended in the manual as an emancipatory concept, an idea that can help workshop participants see that their own assumptions and expectations regarding gender are arbitrary and might be unjust or socially damaging. There is also a hope that, in the intimate space of the workshop, the sharing of participants' own gendered experiences of inequality will inspire greater empathy, perhaps especially in men for women, which will, in turn, facilitate greater critical consciousness about gender.

The handbook explains and illustrates the concepts of gender, gender role stereotypes, and gender-based inequality in multiple ways. For example, it compares breastfeeding as a biological capacity with washing clothes as a gender-based role. And it provides quotations and aphorisms about gender from a range of places around the world, sometimes with explications:

"Men are gold, women are cloth." This expression, which is used as the title of a report on Cambodian attitudes towards sex and HIV, means that women, like a white cloth, are easily soiled by sex . . . whereas men can have repeated sexual experiences and be polished clean, like gold, each time. (PNG NAC 2007, 33)

"I am legally married to my wife and if I have sex with her when she is not ready, that is not rape. A woman is there to serve and dance to the tune of her husband, full stop"—47-year old man in Tanzania. (PNG NAC 2007, 34)

"Women should wear purdah to ensure that innocent men do not get unnecessarily excited by women's bodies and are not unconsciously forced into becoming rapists . . . ."—Malaysian member of Parliament during debate on reform of rape laws. (PNG NAC 2007, 33)

While the written examples regarding gender inequality are taken from all over the world, including wealthy nations such as Canada, the drawn illustrations all depict Papua New Guinean scenarios. They include a bridewealth ceremony, a village scene with women washing clothes and sweeping up the public area, and a man punching his wife while weeping children look on. There is a section that explains the connections between gender roles, gender inequality, and HIV vulnerability by discussing girls' generally lower educational level and access to employment, as well as their lack of power to refuse sex or negotiate safer sex. There are exercises for the participants, with discussion questions about sexual violence (e.g., "Does rape only occur outside of marriage?"; "Are rapists crazy?").

This chapter of the manual covers a wide range of topics in accessible and thought-provoking ways, and while many of the cited statements on gender from around the world might not make much intuitive sense to all Papua New Guinean audiences, they do effectively show that gender inequality is a global issue. More problematically, this chapter of the manual also represents women as oppressed by men, tacitly positioning women and men as antagonists rather than partners. It rhetorically interpellates female participants as victims and creates a space for them to verbalize and share their experiences, but does not create a similar space for male participants. The chapter thus implies that as the dominant gender, men do not experience oppression or marginalization and do not need a space in which to share their gendered or other experiences of inequality.

While embracing the role-plasticity implied by a social constructionist orientation towards gender, Anna also disagreed with some of the specifics in this chapter. She fully supported the idea that women in Papua New Guinea could and should become police officers, pilots, and members of parliament, and she gamely argued, both within and outside the workshop, with Huli men who dismissively mocked this vision of gender equality. She had advocated widely for a bill that would have amended the Papua New Guinea Constitution to reserve twenty-two seats in Parliament for women, and indeed hoped to run for one of these seats (but the bill did not pass). Nevertheless, she also believed that some aspects of biology determined men's and women's behaviors and capacities, though these were not the gendered behaviors and capacities that Western/Northern readers might associate with biological essentialism. For example, she told the participants:

> This manual gets some things wrong. Some things that this handbook says are gender are really sex. God has designed women in a special way. The reason women are able to keep working all day long is because of their wombs. Men do two or three jobs in a day, and they come home hungry and tired. But women keep going and going and going and are never too tired to work. It's because of a certain kind of magic or medicine that they have in their wombs. It gives them strength. Oh no! Look! I'm revealing women's deepest secrets. Well, I'm not giving away the details. But it is true. It is special medicine or magic in women's wombs that gives them so much energy.

This comment was made in response to the group's discussion about the village scene in the handbook. The drawing of women washing clothes and cleaning up the village seems to imply that the disproportionate amount of domestic labor performed by women is a consequence of inequitable gender relations in Papua New Guinea. Anna rebutted this argument by reformulating women's heavy workload as the exercise of their innate, God-given energy, and thus not to be understood as an outcome of male dominance or privilege. In other words, she affirmed a kind of divine biological essentialism, not in order to argue that women were designed or intended for specific *kinds* of labor (indeed, she asserted that women and men were equally able to be loving caregivers for children or MPs), but rather to assert their innate superiority to men in terms of endurance. Women had to do more work, she implied, because men simply did not have the capacity to do so.

It should be noted that Anna seemed determined throughout the workshop to avoid angry confrontation between the male and female participants, and she told me that she believed the most fruitful approach to improving Huli gender relations and to reducing HIV vulnerability was to bring men and women together, not put them in opposition to each other. In other words, where the manual hazardously implied that Papua New Guinea's gendered division of labor might be exploitative, Anna reframed the story as one about gender complementarity and innate female stamina.

Anna's desires to avoid confrontation proved difficult, however. One group exercise, in which the participants were asked to break into same-sex groups and create lists of their respective stereotypical gendered tasks, resulted in angry feelings. In normative Huli discourse, many tasks are said to belong quite rigidly to one or the other gender, so this initially seemed to be a straightforward exercise. When the two groups came back together, the men's list included: dig trenches around family territory, build houses, make bows and arrows, clear land of trees and underbrush for cultivation, plant trees, tribal fighting, build fences, negotiate bridewealth, kill and cook pigs, and cut the cooked pork into proper pieces for distribution. The list created by the women was shorter: give birth and breastfeed; care for pigs, dogs, and children; plant and harvest sweet potatoes; make string bags; and cut and gather the grasses that make the roof of a house. The men's longer list annoyed the women, since they felt that women do more work than men. The men then made the tactical error of pointing out that men make string bags too (which is true, though it tends to be a highly specialized task that only few men do) and asserting that this task should therefore be added to the men's list as well.

The women, now quite provoked, angrily pointed out the difference between dominant discourse and actual practice, by responding that some of the items on the men's list should also go on the women's list. One woman said, "My husband took another wife, and he doesn't come to our household anymore, so I do many of these male tasks myself. I plant and cut down trees, I kill my own pigs, I cut them up and cook them, and I make my own fences." Another added, "My husband left us, and I haven't seen him in years, and so last year I built my own house. I even got up on top and made the roof myself." For women to engage in this last task is traditionally very taboo, and there were a few loud intakes of breath at this assertion, though no one said anything.

At the heart of these women's performances of male tasks, the reader will have noticed, is male absence. As discussed in chapter 3, there is a long history of male outmigration from the Tari area, which has necessitated changes in women's labor, even if this is not reflected in entrenched normative discourse about gender. Moreover, with the more recent influx of money from resource-extraction projects, especially the LNG, there has been an increase in polygamy in some areas (McIlraith et al. 2012), which has similarly caused an increase in de facto female-headed households, as husbands move to reside with their new wives. Thus, in point of fact, many women perform the tasks on the men's list, or, alternatively, they sell garden produce and other goods in order to make money so that they can pay men to do them. Implied by these women's bitterly proud assertions of female self-sufficiency was an angry critique of male absence and male marital privilege.

The women's interjections helped to make Anna's point that many gendered tasks are learned and are therefore not determined by innate sexual characteristics, but they also heightened the tension in the room since everyone knew that it was male neglect, privilege, and abandonment that necessitated these role changes and contributed to the feminization of rural domestic and agricultural labor. Tensions came to a head when one woman proclaimed loudly, followed by angry mutters of agreement from the rest of the women, "Your list subordinates/belittles us women (*List bilong yupela save daunim mipela ol meri*)." The Tok Pisin verb she used, *daunim* (literally, to down someone), can mean either to make someone subservient or to treat them as if they are of lesser value. In other words, she was asserting that by reinscribing normative discourse about gendered tasks, and by creating a long list that made it appear that men did more work than women, the men were discounting women's onerous labor and representing them as less valuable than men.

Recently divorced herself and used to doing some of the tasks on the men's list, Anna in this instance affirmed the women's experiences of forced self-sufficiency and impressed upon the male participants the difficulties faced by female-headed households. In other words, departing somewhat from her earlier assertions about women's greater capacity for work, Anna indicated that this innate, biologically determined stamina was being pressed into excessive service because of social changes such as divorce, increased polygyny, and male out-migration.

Omitting Gender-Based Violence

The most significant and disconcerting way in which Anna deviated from the script of the workshop manual took the form of an omission rather than a reframing or correction of the text: although she covered many of the topics in the chapter about gender, she skipped over the sections on gender inequality and gender-based violence. This is particularly remarkable since repeated surveys and ethnographic research in Papua New Guinea (Toft 1985, Dinnen and Ley 2000, Jolly et al. 2012, Human Rights Watch 2015, Biersack et al. 2016) have shown very high rates of domestic and sexual violence in many areas of the country. Moreover, HIV/AIDS policy documents have repeatedly stressed the connection between gender inequality and HIV vulnerability. For example, the National AIDS Council report, *Papua New Guinea National HIV and AIDS Strategy, 2011–2015,* asserts: "Gender-based violence and sexual violence are endemic in PNG and are a major factor in HIV vulnerability. Interventions which reduce physical and sexual violence against women and girls, and which support survivors of violence, will be urgently scaled-up" (PNG NAC 2010: 34). The U.S. *Papua New Guinea Country Operation Plan (COP) 2016 Strategic Direction Summary* asserts that "Papua New Guinea ranks 140 out of 155 countries in the 2014 Gender Inequality Index," and states that gender-based violence is "one of the greatest barriers to each of the '90: 90: 90' fast track targets" (PEPFAR 2016: 7–8).[2] Demographers and ethnographers of the Huli have also documented a high level of gender violence. Analyzing causes of mortality among the Huli in the 1980s, Peter Geoffrey Barss found very high rates of female homicide, for example, and observed: "The endemic severe violence to adult females appears to be unprecedented for a country not under active attack during time of war" (Barss 1991: chapter 7, p. 29). Because of the area's reputation for violent gender relations, Médecins sans frontières initiated a project in Tari in 2009 dedicated to treating family and sexual violence (MSF 2011). In short, if one were to choose a place in Papua New Guinea where education about gender violence would seem most appropriate, Tari would be high on the list, and Anna's omission of this section of the manual was striking.

But Anna had her reasons. She explained to me later that she had been worried that a discussion of gender violence might antagonize the male participants. They could quit the workshop or even shut it down if they so chose. She also wanted to avoid a workshop dynamic in which the female participants heaped blame upon

r violent marital relations, because of the possible repercussions afterwards:
not want the workshop to be the cause of lasting ill will between any of
the participants, and she herself did not want to become known as someone who
exacerbated marital conflict by encouraging bitterness and resentment.

Equally important, she disagreed with the manual's way of interpellating participants as gendered subjects—especially things like the drawing of the man
punching his wife, which depicted men as aggressors and women as victims
(cf. Merry 2006). And she deliberately countered this rhetorical strategy of the
manual through her own assertions that emphasized agency on the part of both
genders. For example, in the one instance in which she did mention gender-based
violence—in her discussion of rape as one possible mode of HIV transmission—she
asserted that men rape women, but equally that women rape men. By this
she meant that some women seduce men and deliberately try to undermine their
resolve to be faithful to their wives. Both acts, she felt, were forms of aggression
that intentionally removed the capacity of the target to refuse sex. She did not
think that they were equal forms of aggression—victims of rape often suffered
from shock and other injuries—but she was unhappy that only one of these forms
of aggression was addressed in the manual. Her critique suggests that the manual's
authors do not fully understand how sexual aggression is understood in various
areas of Papua New Guinea, nor do they comprehend the logic of gender complementarity, which assumes that both men and women have agentival capacities.

In short, Anna skimmed the sections on gender inequality and skipped the
sections on gender-based violence not only because they were fraught topics that
might destabilize the workshop, but also because she felt that the manual simpli-
fied highly complex issues and reduced men and women to two-dimensional figures, in which men were fully agentive and culpable, and women were not. "After
all," she told me, "it's true that men hit their wives, but it's also true that women
hit or even stab their husbands. And women, when they are angry, also tell their
husbands that they are worthless trash, and this is a cause of fighting. Maybe we
Huli hit each other too much, but the bigger problems are that money is short, and
husbands and wives don't know how to talk to each other well."

Anna's skeptical appraisal of the manual resonates to some extent with African
and other non-Western feminist critiques of white feminist interventions on
behalf of women in postcolonial contexts. Many of these scholars have pointed
out the ways in which white feminist discourses about "third world women" often
represent them as victims, emphasize male violence against women while obscur-
ing other issues pertinent to women, assume that some customs are imposed
by men upon women and are manifestations of their dominance, and willfully
ignore the imperialist histories that undermined women's authority in precolonial
societies (Mohanty 1984, Amadiume 1987, Mama 1997, Oyewumi 1997).

These scholars also note that white feminists often problematically presume
that the epistemologies and strategies that have informed feminist movements in

the West are the "right" ones and should be adopted globally, ignoring the possibility of alternative philosophies of gender and social action. For example, Philomena Steady, a Sierra Leonean anthropologist, has argued that Western feminism, much like Western liberal humanism more generally, is animated by and organizes itself around concepts of individual autonomy, gender dichotomy, and opposition, while African feminism, in contrast, is organized around the values of gender complementarity and social communalism (Steady 1987; see also Oyewumi 1997). "The language of feminist engagement in Africa (collaborate, negotiate, compromise) runs counter to the language of Western feminist scholarship and engagement (challenge, disrupt, deconstruct, blow apart, etc.)," Obioma Nnaemeka writes. "African feminism challenges through negotiation, accommodation, and compromise" (Nnaemeka 2004: 380). From this perspective, the AIDS workshop manual could be viewed as inspired by a white Western/Northern feminist orientation, in which men and women are adversaries, with men imposing their power through violence. Anna's approach, in contrast, was informed by a philosophy of gender complementarity and collaboration, and she silenced those sections of the manual that assumed and encouraged gendered subject formation based on antagonism.

JENDA AS MORAL WORK ON THE SELF

As indicated in her observation above that wives play their part in marital violence by, for example, disparaging their husbands as worthless, or by engaging in physical violence themselves, gendered conflict was not just about agency for Anna, but also about culpability, which is to say that it was also about morality. In other words, according to Anna, in many if not all instances, wives as well as husbands said or did something to humiliate or enrage their spouses, actions that were both hurtful and indicative of a need for moral self-reflection and work on the self. From her perspective, it was the rare case in which the *tene* (root or cause) of marital conflict was singular and locatable in only one spouse's behavior. Fighting or HIV transmission between spouses was a consequence of larger moral problems within a marriage. The key to prevention was thus cultivation of moral improvement, not cultivation of a critical consciousness about gender, as the authors of the workshop manual might have it. At one point during the workshop, Anna therefore articulated her mission not as narrowly focused on HIV prevention, but more broadly on joining men and women together in a shared project of individual, marital, and cultural moral betterment (see also Wardlow 2012).

Jenda—conceptualized as the ability to become a better man or woman—was at the center of her pedagogy. Departing significantly from the workshop manual, Anna's explication of *jenda* oscillated between being gender—that is, a category that she contrasted with sex and explained as the learned behaviors associated with being male or female—and being something that was completely untethered from biological sex, and was instead a site for ethical work on the self. To illustrate, below are ways in which Anna defined or explained *jenda*, and, in some instances, its difference from sex. As the reader will see, *jenda* is sometimes juxtaposed to sex, is sometimes almost entirely sex-free, and is sometimes somewhere in between:

"*Jenda* is what you learn on your life's journey."

"*Jenda* is important because you can change it. If you are sinful, you can become a religious man. If you are a woman who plays cards, you can change and become a woman who plants sweet potatoes. *Jenda* is the things you can change about yourself."

"*Jenda* is learned things—our behaviors, the thoughts we think, the food we make. Can we change these things? [The participants responded: "Yes!"] Sex is different. God designed us in a particular way. Women are always women. Men are always men."

"*Jenda* is our ability to change our behavior. *Jenda* is when you are a man who drinks, and you decide to stop being a drinker. Or, when you are a man who participates in tribal fighting, and you decide not to participate in tribal fighting any more. *Jenda* tells us that we can change, so change! We all need to change, so that as a society we can avoid troubles like tribal fighting, drinking, and HIV/AIDS."

"I can't feed my baby beard hair to make her grow a beard and become a man. She is a girl. This won't change. That is sex. *Jenda* is what you learn in life that gives you power. For example, you learn to be a pilot or you learn to be a nurse."

In these examples, *jenda* has an unfixed relationship to biological sex: sometimes it refers to the social roles that sexed bodies come to play, but more often Anna used the concept of *jenda* to encourage the participants to reflect on their socially or self-destructive practices and to agree that moral improvement was possible and would contribute to the betterment of Huli marriages and Huli society.

Anna also explained *jenda* as an aspirational pathway—that is, a "journey" through which one might learn valuable knowledge and accrue skills that could "give one power." This understanding of *jenda* was perhaps inspired by the somewhat misguided examples in the handbook of gender-stereotyped jobs, such as nurses and pilots. In Papua New Guinea, while nurses and pilots are, indeed, gender-stereotyped jobs, they are also careers that are near impossible for most people to obtain. In other words, they are also class-stereotyped jobs. Few children complete grade school, let alone high school or any tertiary education, so any of the workshop participants would have been overjoyed if their children (of either gender) became a nurse or pilot. Thus, as Anna and the participants understood these examples, *jenda* was not about rigidly entrenched and constraining gender roles, but rather about the possibilities of upward class mobility for a person who dedicated him or herself to accumulating valuable skills and to abstaining from self-defeating habits and behaviors, such as gambling or drinking. In short, Anna took from the manual the idea that gender is that which "is learned" or "can be changed," and put it to work as an agent of hope, moral uplift, and progress.

This is not to say that *jenda* was completely unlinked from a notion of gender as learned and expected sex role. Anna also deployed her concept of *jenda* to introduce the idea that spouses should consider and openly communicate about gender role flexibility in marriage. As she explained it:

> What each couple needs to do is figure out what they specialize in. That's *jenda*. If the wife is not a specialist in cooking, her husband should help her, and not get angry. He should not assume she is an expert in cooking just because she is a woman. Maybe she never learned to cook—that's *jenda*. Or me, I'm an expert in cutting up roasted pigs and distributing the pieces appropriately. I know that men usually do this job, but I'm very good at it, better than my husband, so I do this in my family.

Here, *jenda*—used by Anna to mean both culturally defined gendered social roles and individuals' innate, but changeable, skills, habits, and propensities—creates a context in which a husband might be willing to abdicate a prestigious social role (e.g., cutting up a roasted pig and distributing the portions to guests) if his wife happens to be more adept at the task. Both male privilege and female duty, are, to some extent, subtly redefined here as gender-free talents or aptitudes. The concept of *jenda*, as explained by Anna, is an emancipatory and empowering one, but it operates by creating a space where husbands and wives can discuss their aptitudes and rearrange their tasks accordingly, rather than abide by rigid customary roles. Also notable here is Anna's attempt to guide the workshop participants in one aspect of building a companionate marriage—that is, by setting aside customary dictates and instead verbally negotiating which spouse will do what tasks.

THE RETURN OF THE REPRESSED:
GENDER CONFLICT ERUPTS

Anna's attempts to recruit the participants into *jenda* as a modern, aspirational, moral project did not completely succeed in containing or silencing gender inequality in the workshop. The gender-role list-making session was just one of a number of moments when the participants became upset. On the second day, a male clinician working in the region, but from another area of Papua New Guinea, came to the workshop to speak to the participants about sexual health. He was nervous, and perhaps that explains why his presentation quickly devolved into an emotional outburst about Huli women's lack of sexual hygiene. The number of Huli women he had examined who had severe, untreated, and foul-smelling vaginal infections was awful, he told the participants; he had never seen anything like it in his previous assignments. His disgust and distress were plain. His speech sped up and rose in pitch. The participants all looked at the floor, but I could see that some faces expressed embarrassment, anger, or revulsion. His repeated mention of the foul-smelling vaginal discharge he encountered seemed to paralyze them. "You

Huli women," he concluded, "you need to learn to wash better after sex." Finally the session ended and we broke for tea.

Drawing on Foucault, Charles Briggs has argued that authoritative biomedical knowledge is a powerful mode of governmentality, shaping individual conduct, producing health-oriented subjectivities, and defining citizenship in relation to this authoritative knowledge:

> [H]ealth becomes an ethical imperative, requiring individuals to regulate their behavior and reshape their selves in keeping with new medical knowledge. Those who seem to succeed acquire the status of sanitary citizens . . . individuals deemed to possess modern medical understandings of the body, health, and illness, practice hygiene, and depend on doctors and nurses when they are sick. . . . People who are judged to be incapable of adopting this modern medical relationship to the body, hygiene, illness, and healing—or who refuse to do so—become unsanitary subjects. (Briggs 2005: 272; see also Briggs with Mantini-Briggs 2004)

This knowledge is unevenly distributed, with some actors designated as "producers of knowledge, others like translators and disseminators, others like receivers, and some simply out of the game" (Briggs 2005: 274; see also Andersen 2017).

Thus far, the female participants in the workshop with their male counterparts had embodied the role of "receivers," a role that positioned them comfortably on the path to sanitary citizenship. Indeed, arguably this is one function of AIDS awareness and other health-related workshops: to select members of an unsanitary subject demographic, offer them the possibility of improving their position in relation to authoritative biomedical knowledge, and thereby hold out the promise of sanitary citizenship and the privileges it confers. But when the male health worker addressed the female participants as "You Huli women" and attributed his caseload of sexual health problems to their lack of hygiene, they were abruptly evicted from sanitary citizenship. In other words, sanitary citizenship was not only ethnicized, with the Huli singled out as less hygienic than other cultural groups, but also gendered. Sitting side by side, receiving the same biomedical knowledge, it was the women, not the men, who were scolded as dirty and ignorant.

I found myself, sitting on the floor, legs crossed, feeling suddenly too aware of my own genitals, wondering if other women in the room were feeling that way too, and thinking about the many times I've experienced yeast infections in Papua New Guinea because my underwear wouldn't dry during the rainy season or because the guesthouse's water tank was broken, and it was hard to stay clean. And then I thought about sex and women's lesser control over when it happens, and how difficult it would be to wash afterwards if you lived in a bush house with no running water and you weren't willing to stumble down to the nearest stream in the middle of the night. And then I thought that the health worker, without any laboratory facilities, had no means of precisely diagnosing the infections he encountered, and that many of them were likely transmitted sexually to his female patients from their husbands, and no amount of washing after sex was going to prevent those.

Indeed, it is worth pointing out that this instance of producing an ethnicized and gendered unsanitary subject was based on the deployment of *inaccurate* biomedical knowledge. Much as Briggs suggests, it was the health worker's designation as an implementer and disseminator of biomedical knowledge, and his clearly superior standing as a sanitary citizen, that authorized his flawed and biased usage of this knowledge. In short, I thought about how gender inequality intersects with lack of sanitation infrastructure and female reproductive physiology to produce sexually transmitted infections in women, who were then rebuked as diseased, dirty, and irresponsible in front of their male community leader peers. It was, for me, and I suspect for many of the female participants (who, uncharacteristically, were completely silent during the tea break), a humiliating gendered moment, not a *jenda* moment.

Gender inequality created "ugly feelings" (Ngai 2007) in the workshop again on the fourth day, shortly after the gender-role list-making exercise. One of the male participants rather sanctimoniously announced that one health issue they hadn't discussed yet was women's practice of handing off their babies to other women. "We men don't like that." There was silence. And then one woman responded carefully, "Sometimes we have to hand our baby to another woman if there's something we need to do—like buy something at the market. Sometimes we can't carry a baby and do other things at the same time." "But you don't know what diseases those women might have. It is really unhealthy for you to hand our babies to other women." More silence. Then another woman quite testily said, "Well, if you men would agree to carry your own babies, we wouldn't have to worry about that." "But this is against Huli custom. You know that men do not carry babies. It is unhealthy." "No one believes that anymore. You men carry your babies when you are at home. You just don't want to do it in public because you worry that other men will make fun of you and gossip that you are acting like a woman." "Yes," another man interjected angrily, "this is true. How would it look if a man is carrying his young children while his wife walks around with her hands free as if she is the man? And most of the time you women don't have something you need to do—you just want to go talk and laugh with your friends." "And that's not a good reason?!" "No, that's not a good reason!" As one might imagine, the participants' voices became louder and angrier.

Anna jumped in to assert that her husband had often carried their young children if she had specific things she needed to buy at the market, but the participants talked over her and began yelling. Anna tried to bring things to a close with another comment about *jenda*, and how this was another example of how couples needed to decide together which customs to follow and how to allocate various household responsibilities. But most of the men were adamant that how a man was perceived by his peers—and especially being perceived as appropriately masculine by having his hands free and not being feminized by childcare—took precedence over other considerations, because it could affect his political and economic relations with other men. The women remained adamant that if men were not willing to carry their own children in public, they would continue to hand them over to female friends as they saw fit.

I was nonplussed. This was what made the participants most upset—so upset that they were yelling at each other? Not the male and female condom demonstrations? Not the discussions about men marrying multiple wives and still engaging in extramarital sex?

This impromptu discussion had escalated into such a vociferous argument, some participants explained to me, because (1) the men seemed to feel no compunction about taking control of the space of the workshop to chastise the women, and (2) this touched on a number of other issues: men's general disapproval of women's friendships, and their attempts to limit them (Wardlow 2006a); men's attempts to use women's childcare responsibilities to limit and control their freedom of movement; and women's impatience with men's unwillingness to be seen performing domestic roles in public, thus burdening women with stressful multitasking. In other words, this issue affected women's labor, autonomy, and sociality. Since men refused to undertake childcare in the public domain, women felt that they had no right to comment on how women managed their many responsibilities.

CONCLUSION

Discussing humanitarian organizations' medicalization of wartime sexual violence, Miriam Ticktin observes,

> Gender relations are relations of power. As both an analytic category and a social process, gender is relational—it has no meaning or existence alone . . . gender relations might be relations of domination or subordination, or of mutual respect or interdependence. Whatever the nature of these relations, when we speak of gender-based violence, we imply relations of power. (Ticktin 2011: 254)

Something similar might be said about HIV/AIDS: that when we speak of HIV/ AIDS, we imply relations of power—relations of power that produce gender as difference, category, and experience, thereby creating differences in HIV vulnerability. And yet this is not how gender is explained in the workshop manual. Instead, although attempting to tackle the issues of gender-based inequality and gender-based violence, the manual relies on a dated social-constructionist conceptualization of gender, which is defined simply as "learned attributes and behaviors" that "can be changed" (p. 30). Indeed, some sections of this chapter in the manual can be read as artifacts of anthropological work: anthropology may have questioned and moved beyond a social-constructionist conceptualization of gender, but it clearly has lasting life as an element of health and development projects.

It was this social-constructionist aspect of the manual, I believe, that created some of the challenges that Anna had to navigate. Gender explained as a relation of power embedded in a matrix of other relations of power (employed/jobless, employer/employee, former colonial ruler/former colonial subject, landowner/non-landowner, white/black, urban/rural, educated/uneducated) might have created a conceptual space in which the participants could talk about gendered inequality and violence as intersecting with and shaped by other relations of inequality and violence. And this kind of framework—one that recognized men's experiences of humiliation, fear, marginalization, and violence—might have made a discussion of gender-based violence less threatening and more viable. But gender inequality in the manual is presented as women's inequality, without any contextualization regarding men's history of colonial and postcolonial oppression or marginalization. Similarly, the manual takes an ahistorical approach to gender: nowhere does it ask participants to reflect on and discuss how relations between men and women have changed, why, and with what consequences. The manual's ahistorical approach (presumably based on a notion of "culture" as bounded and unchanging) is perhaps especially problematic in a region where such profound socioeconomic changes have occurred, all of which impact gender relations. Thus, Anna was equipped only with a notion of gender as learned and changeable behavior, and she was then expected to lead a discussion about gender-based violence cued by drawings that interpellated female participants as victims of violence, and male participants as the perpetrators. It is not surprising that she declined to embark on this discussion.

The other, related challenge created by the manual was its implicit positioning of men and women as adversaries rather than partners—for example, in the manual's litany of disparaging quotations and aphorisms about gender and its illustration of marital conflict with a drawing of a man punching a collapsing woman, whose eyes are shut. While the intent of these discursive strategies is surely to convey that male dominance is a global issue, and not something that Papua New Guinean women should feel alone in experiencing, the manual seems very much informed by a Northern liberal feminism in which the genders are locked into an antagonistic relationship and, as Saba Mahmood puts it, female agency "is conceptualized on the binary model of subordination and subversion" (Mahmood 2005: 14). In other words, the presumed female sociopolitical subject is an individual whose autonomy is either subordinated by patriarchy or oriented towards subverting it; her agency can either reinforce or resist male dominance, a conceptualization that leaves little space or legitimacy for other intentions, such as cooperation or negotiation between the genders.

Drawing on her own convictions about how best to improve troubled Huli marital relations—an aim she agreed with—Anna resisted this more binary and antagonistic model in the manual, and formulated her own—*jenda*—which positioned men and women as having shared (though perhaps not equal) culpability in the creation of conflict, and shared responsibility for the work of improving marital relations. Here it is important to observe the influential role that workshop educators can play in the health knowledge economy: in Briggs's scheme, they are positioned as disseminators, tasked with informing target audiences about public health knowledge so that it might change their behavior. However, they are also sometimes certain that the scripted strategies for achieving certain goals are wrongheaded, and so, exercising translational agency, they may alter, silence, or speak back to this knowledge. Thus, Anna took the manual's behavior-change approach—an approach criticized ad nauseam by anthropologists—and appropriated it to urge the participants to work ethically on themselves for the sake of Huli society.

Anna's attempts to recruit the participants to the concept of *jenda* were only partially successful, however. Women's subordination was reproduced in the workshop (e.g., when the clinician scolded the women, not the men, about sexual hygiene), and anger about male privileges (to marry polygynously, to walk "hands free" in public, to publicly chastise women) rose to the surface and erupted sporadically. Huli marital relations are, in fact, often marked by strife, and listing gender-stereotyped tasks is not going to go very far in confronting the distressing dimensions of marriage. A more intersectional approach that enabled participants to discuss gender relations in the context of other relations of power and inequality might better enable participants to engage in challenging and painful discussions.

5

Caring for the Self

HIV and Emotional Regulation

Recall Last Minute Lucy from chapter 2, who had been infected with HIV "at the last minute" (that is, when she had reached the age when women's sexual activity is expected to end). After many years of living in her eldest brother's household, she had left in anger after an altercation with him, and gone home with a man she met at a *dawe anda*. It was through this relationship that she was infected with HIV. When her eldest brother learned she was HIV-positive he refused to have anything to do with her. She had eventually given up trying to mend their relationship and now avoided him because of the negative feelings he caused her to have:

> My brother's family has caused me a lot of worry. [How so?] They don't take care of me, and they gossip about me, and say things like "At the last minute she took her old lady vagina out and fucked around, and look what happened. She got AIDS." My brother has said this to me in front of other people. And this makes me angry. And it makes me worry. And when I am worried I develop lots of these little sores (she pointed to dozens of small ulcers on her lower legs), and the skin around my eyes turns black, and my eyes are red for no reason. . . . When we were children our mother ran away and married another man, so I became like the mother to my younger siblings. I was the oldest girl, and so I walked them to school, I cooked for them. I wanted to continue going to school myself, but I became a replacement for my mother, and I had to stay home. And my eldest brother used to feel compassion for me. He remembered all I had done for him when he was little, and he was generous to me. When my husband beat me, he would take me in and demand compensation. But now when we see each other on the road he looks the other way (*em pulim nus*). I'm ashamed to run into him because he treats me so poorly in front of other people.

Lucy, like many of the women I interviewed, drew direct connections between experiencing intense negative emotions and bodily symptoms of illness, such as sores, changes in skin color or hair texture, rashes, respiratory infections, and malaria. Fearing that intense feelings of anger, shame, and worry would "wake up the virus" or would reduce the effectiveness of their antiretroviral medication (ARVs) by blocking pathways within the body, many avoided people and situations that might trigger these feelings. They also developed personal strategies for trying to regulate their emotions, striving for greater equanimity, always in the hope that their ARVs would work best, and that the virus would remain "asleep" or "fenced in by the medicine" if they could keep themselves from feeling "bad" emotions.

Women's experiences of being HIV-positive varied immensely. A few women I interviewed were essentially homeless, having been evicted by family, one even traveling from one relative to another with a thick, plastic tarp, so that she could sleep outside in their fields with their permission. In contrast, a few women said that they were happier than they had ever been before. Nevertheless, despite differences in age, marital and reproductive history, and family acceptance (or not), they shared a number of characteristics, one of which was that emotional regulation was a key component of their self-care.

The women I interviewed were, on average, an older group than has been typical of much research about HIV, and this surely informed some of their opinions and attitudes, particularly about marriage, which I discuss near the end of the chapter. Twenty of the thirty women fell roughly into the middle-aged and older category; nine were in their twenties or early thirties and had young children; and one was a teenager. Thirteen of the women were widows (their husbands had all died of AIDS-related illnesses); ten were effectively divorced (they had either run away from or been abandoned by their husbands); three were currently married; and four had never married. And, as mentioned in earlier chapters, between twenty-two and twenty-five of them had been infected with HIV by their husbands.

A TALE OF TWO CLINICS

In 2012 and 2013, when I interviewed people receiving care for HIV, patients in the Tari area had a choice of two clinics—one was based in Tari District Hospital, in the center of Tari town; the other was located behind the large Catholic church just outside of town. The hospital clinic underwent the most change over the course of my research. In 2004, the nurse running the clinic showed me the records she kept of HIV-positive patients, and spoke of how demoralizing it was to keep these records, knowing there was little she could do to help them. At that time there was no rapid testing at the hospital, and there were no ARVs in any case. By 2013, however, the Oil Search Health Foundation had taken over the management of the clinic, upgrading the building facilities, hiring many additional staff, improving record-keeping, and providing vehicles for community outreach and the support of a number of satellite clinics. And, being based at the hospital, this clinic was able to refer patients for X-rays and laboratory tests for other diseases, like TB or malaria. The waiting room was usually full, sometimes with lines out the door, and the clinic often had a frenetic feel to it.

The AIDS Care Centre run by the Catholic Church, in contrast, was a calm oasis. Behind and hidden from the road by a large church, it rarely had more than ten patients in it at one time, and if the benches in the waiting room were full, patients could rest on the plentiful areas of shady grass outside. Most of the patients weren't Catholic; the clinic served anyone who wanted HIV testing or treatment and didn't ask about religion. The staff also had a reputation for being less judgmental than those at the Tari District Hospital clinic. They all chewed betel nut on breaks, and two of them smoked cigarettes, which perhaps accounted for their reluctance to rebuke patients for doing so, even though they knew that abstaining was strongly advised for people living with HIV. Other than these differences, the two clinics were very similar in terms of the counselling they provided to patients regarding self-care, adherence to the ART regimen, disclosing their HIV status to spouses and family members, and abstaining from extramarital sex.

The two clinics had both a cooperative and somewhat competitive relationship. The Care Centre only provided treatment for HIV, sexually transmitted infections, and some opportunistic infections. There were no laboratory facilities, so it referred some patients to the hospital, particularly when it suspected TB. Some of the hospital clinic staff hinted that the Catholic clinic was unnecessary; after all, they said, it was only a short distance away and patients could just as easily come to the hospital. Moreover, and more important, they asserted that it "confused" their records and statistics when they did lab tests or X-rays for patients who weren't registered with them. My decoding of these assertions was that while this probably did make record-keeping more onerous, the larger issue was that the two clinics were competing for patients, and the hospital staff were irked at having to provide care for patients who couldn't be counted in the reports they submitted to the Global Fund, the Health Department, and the National AIDS Council, because these patients had been tested and were receiving ARVs from the Care Centre. For their part, the staff at the Catholic clinic occasionally expressed discontent that the hospital clinic staff, as government employees, had more access to in-service training and professional development opportunities.

POST-DIAGNOSIS LIFE

The women I interviewed expressed profound gratitude for their medication. Most of them had known people—husbands in most instances, brothers or sisters for a few—who had died of AIDS-related illnesses before ARVs became available in Tari. Many said things like, "It came too late for my husband. The medicine became available just a few months after he died, but it came in time to save my life." Knowing that ARVs were keeping them alive generated an affectively intense form of attachment to their medication: many referred to their medication as

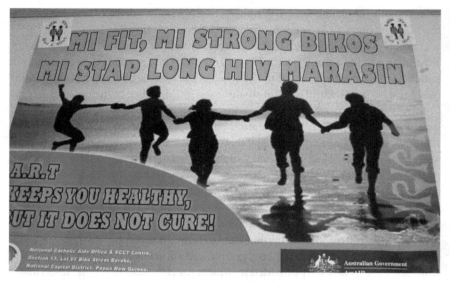

FIGURE 7. Poster inside a health center: "I am fit and strong because I take HIV medicine." Photo by author.

"my life," "my husband now" (meaning that ARVs were now what protected a woman), or "my bones" (the Tok Pisin word *bun* means bone(s), but is also used to mean staple food or that which is a necessity or is held very dearly). One woman declared, "This medicine is my husband, my mommy, and my army [*man bilong mi, mommy bilong mi, na army bilong mi*]." Rather than keeping their supply at home, most women carried it around with them in their string bags. Some simply felt reassured knowing that their medicine was on their person rather than some distance off. Others feared that a pending tribal fight or lack of money might prevent them from reaching home, which meant that they wanted their medication with them at all times. And, still others wanted to be able to display their medications as evidence of their HIV-positive status, should a man proposition them too aggressively, something I discuss in the next chapter.

While profoundly grateful for their continued lives, many women also articulated uncertainty and discomfort about the degree of dependence created by the daily regimen of taking ARVs. During one period of doing interviews in 2012, because of a countrywide shortage, most of the women had been without ARVs for three months; a few had begun experiencing breakdowns in health, including repeated malaria, respiratory infections, and skin ulcers. The possibility that the drugs might never be replenished, or that they might stop working sometime in the future, concerned all the women. Almost all of them said they had known people who had been taking ARVs but died nonetheless. A few said that these people had started taking the medicines too late or had taken them irregularly; in other words, they put forward plausible explanations for why the ARVs had not worked as they were supposed to. For most, however, it remained a mystery why the drugs had failed, and this made them feel vulnerable to a similar fate, even after years of thriving on the medicines. Living on ARVs was, they seemed to suggest, like living in a subjunctive, rather than an indicative, state—tenuous, conditional, steeped in both yearning and regret. The perpetual uncertainty about the reliable supply of ARVS, or their long-term efficacy, motivated vigilant self-scrutiny about their own self-care.

The post-diagnosis lives of the women I interviewed varied significantly, and much depended on how their natal families responded to their HIV-positive diagnosis. Compare, for example, the experiences of Gloria and Shelly.

Gloria left school in grade three in order to help her family pan for gold during the Mt. Kare gold rush in 1988. She married a man she met at Mt. Kare, whom she described as a criminal who had many sexual partners and run-ins with the police. Around 2005, noticing that he was losing weight and was constantly unwell, she began to suspect he might have AIDS:

> When I asked him about it, he said it was a result of the police shooting him before— that his injuries had never healed and they were making him constantly ill. But I believed that he had AIDS. [Did you tell him this?] No, I locked it in my mind and didn't talk about it.... He was diagnosed in 2006, before treatment became available, and died that same year.

In 2007, Gloria herself tested positive, began taking ARVs, and had flourished:

> Now my house is bigger and nicer than other people's houses. And I have more pigs than other people. I take care of chickens and ducks. I grow things in the garden. The way I live now is completely different from how I lived with my husband. Now I take care of myself, and I live better than when I lived with him. I travel by myself up and down the highway, and find little things to sell to make money.... I live with my mother. She's old, and I take care of her. And sometimes my younger brother lives with us. He doesn't have a job, so I take care of him too.

Gloria's life improved after being diagnosed with HIV and initiating treatment, though, perhaps more to the point, her life improved after her husband died and her HIV-positive status enabled her to move back to her parents' home. She described herself as profoundly happier than when she was married.

Gloria's ability to thrive was made possible by a number of circumstances. First, she responded very well to the medication, and said she never experienced fatigue or any other symptoms that might prevent her from doing a lot of physical labor. Second, her success at farming and making money through small sales had put her in the enviable position of being able to help others, even those who might otherwise have been tempted to treat her badly:

> People know my reputation. They know that if they have no money or pigs and they need some, they can come to me and I will help them. So they think to themselves, "She's a sick woman. She has this sickness. If we hit her or do something and she dies,

who can we rely on to help us?" So no one wants to hurt me or insult me. They try to make me happy—they greet me on the road and shake my hand. If they see me sitting alone, they come over and talk to me.

In other words, people in her community, without openly acknowledging her HIV-positive status, demonstrated their acceptance of her by making a point of speaking to and touching her. She was aware, however, that this might not have been the case if she weren't in a position to help others with their children's school fees or bridewealth payments. Finally, her family recognized her as the victim of her husband's extramarital liaisons: they had approved of him when he asked to marry her, because he had helped them pan for gold at Mt. Kare; they admired her loyalty to him as his wife, even in the face of his sexual license and criminal exploits; but they blamed him for her HIV-positive status. From their perspective, she had married appropriately (that is, with their approval) and had been a good wife (even though it turned out badly), and her reputation was therefore sound. Thus, they were happy to take her back when he died.

This was not the case for approximately one-third of the women I interviewed, and a woman's reputation pre-diagnosis often determined how her family would respond to her post-diagnosis. A family's response, in turn, strongly shaped how a woman fared. Shelly, for example, asserted that she had been rebellious when she was younger, had married her husband without her family's permission, and had lived in urban areas away from Tari (that is, in environments considered morally corrupting). Her two older brothers believed that she was the one who had strayed sexually and infected her husband. She admitted that this was, in fact, possible, but that it was unlikely, because her husband had known he was HIV-positive and didn't tell her. After her first two children died when they were babies and she developed sores on her breasts, she sought medical help, tested HIV-positive, and was told to bring her husband for testing:

And he too tested positive. But then I found out that he already knew that he was HIV-positive and had been taking medicine [He already knew?!] Yes, he tricked me. He pretended he didn't know, and he went for another test, but he knew, and he had been taking medicine for a year.

Unhappy with the antiretroviral regimen and unwilling to give up his pre-diagnosis way of life, her husband stopped taking his ARVs, Shelly said, and he died in 2009: "I started taking the medicine, and I had my third baby, and he's still alive. My husband died when I was pregnant."

Her family refused to take her in, however:

My family yelled at me and called me an AIDS woman in public. They wouldn't take me in—they evicted me, they insulted me, they hit me, they told everyone I had AIDS, they cut me with a bush knife (she showed me a large scar on her shoulder), and forced me out. They said, "You yourself found this sickness. Where you found it, we don't know, but you have it and you brought it back here. Take it away. You cannot live here."

Desperate, but also furious and humiliated, Shelly responded by exchanging sex for money:

> They called me an AIDS woman in public, so I thought to myself, "Fine. You say I'm an AIDS woman, then I will act like an AIDS woman, and go around on the road." That's how I got this baby (her fourth, an infant on her lap when I interviewed her in 2012). [So do you passenger around to make money and take care of yourself?] Yes. [And when you do this, do you tell the men?] Yes, usually I tell them. And once I found a man who was also HIV-positive and I stayed with him for a while. When I was passengering around for money I tried to find men who were also HIV-positive, not normal men. But this is very hard. I didn't want to infect other people, but I had to find a way to get money. (Here her voice suggested irritated embarrassment so I changed the subject.)

Ostracized by her family, Shelly was homeless when I met her:

> Sometimes I sleep in people's pig houses (small structures for pigs, normally not tall enough for a person to stand up in). I carry a mosquito net with me and I hang it over the house and make a small fire for my children. [Your family's pig house?] No, other people's pig houses. Anyone who will let me stay. And for a while I had a tarp I could make a tent out of. And sometimes people are sorry for me and they invite me to come stay with them. An aunty lets me stay in her house sometimes.

Gloria and Shelly represent two extremes on a continuum of post-diagnosis well-being: unlike Gloria, most of the women were not better off economically than they had been pre-diagnosis, but, unlike Shelly, most of the other women had places to live, even if they felt that they were at the mercy of kin who might evict them if they caused "trouble" (discussed in the next chapter).

ANTIRETROVIRAL ADHERENCE

The women I interviewed spoke of a range of practices of self-care. The most important of these was acknowledging that "ART has its own laws [*em igat lo bilong em*]." These "laws," as Louise Rasmussen observes, comprise "a set of rules that are defined as central to achieving good treatment outcomes and preventing the spread of HIV" (Rasmussen 2014: 257). First and foremost, of course, is adherence to the antiretroviral regimen, which requires taking one or more pills, precisely twelve hours apart, at the same times every day. In addition, patients should strive to eat a healthy diet, with plenty of protein and fresh fruits and vegetables, while abstaining from overwork, alcohol, and smoking. They are also expected to avoid sex without condoms (unless, following consultation, they are trying to get pregnant), and the health workers at both clinics in Tari often urged patients to avoid sex altogether, telling them that the "heat" and strong sensations caused by sex would "wake up" or "strengthen" the virus. A few of the health workers who were from the Tari area also drew on Huli conceptualizations of sex as a meeting or confrontation between the different bloods of two people, with one partner's blood inevitably being stronger than the other's. If the patient's blood was stronger, they said, there was a greater risk that she might infect her sexual partner; if her sexual partner's blood was stronger, it could wake up the virus and make it more virulent. Given these two bad outcomes, they implied that sex was best avoided.

Much of the existing anthropological literature has emphasized the governmental and disciplinary effects of the ARV adherence counselling provided by health workers. For example, Vinh-Kim Nguyen (2013), highlighting historical links between religious institutions and AIDS NGOs in their elicitation of personal narratives about sex, analyzes HIV counselling as a "confessional technology" that works to produce a patient-subject who is "empowered" to live a morally responsible life, and persuaded that the revelation of the self's sexual secrets to a counsellor is crucial for the unfolding of this empowerment. Dominik Mattes, writing of Tanzanian HIV patients, asserts that medical authorities endeavor "to extensively modify [patients'] conduct, ways of thinking, and social interactions toward what is considered 'appropriate' and 'healthy'" with the aim of producing "an obedient and self-responsible patient" (Mattes 2011: 160). To that end, the HIV-care establishment in Tanzania engages in a range of practices that Mattes sums up as "the system of adherence production" (162), which includes: mandatory attendance at three adherence education classes in the company of a treatment supporter, and instilling in patients the concept of ARVs as "a lifelong contract" in which continued access to treatment requires obeying health workers' instructions. "Ironically, their 'self-responsibility' in the sense of adhering to the treatment regime was established through a rigid control system that favored their disempowerment, with mechanisms of stimulus and punishment aimed at their full subjugation to medical authorities," Mattes concludes (2011:177, see also Rasmussen 2014, Hardon 2012, Burchardt 2014).

To some extent these scholars' insights apply to the situation in Tari. On occasion (though certainly not consistently) I heard clinic staff inform newly diagnosed patients that it was their duty to adhere to the antiretroviral regime because "foreign donors have made these drugs available to you. The Papua New Guinea government isn't paying for these drugs. Other countries, because they are sorry for people in Papua New Guinea, are paying for these medicines. So be reliable, don't waste them, don't be defiant." In other words, they attempted to discipline patients by incorporating them into a global biomedical-moral assemblage in which the pity felt by the foreign donor for the distant, suffering other motivated a life-saving gift that had to be repaid through dutiful compliance. However, it should be noted that after treatment initiation, HIV-positive patients in Tari typically only saw health workers once every three months in order to pick up their next supply of medication. If they reported good health and no adverse side effects, these appointments were often quite short, and staff never made home visits.

Moreover, unlike the sites discussed by the above scholars, patients in Tari were never threatened with treatment discontinuation for noncompliant behaviour. And, although patients were supposed to bring a treatment supporter to their first appointment, some of them didn't, and the staff initiated their treatment anyway, knowing full well that they might not have disclosed their status to family and that they might not have the social support thought to be important for treatment adherence. Furthermore, all of the above scholars emphasize the importance of AIDS support groups in reinforcing clinical disciplinary practices. As Ruth Prince argues, "Support groups are places where the pharmaceutical regime of the clinic meets the humanitarian economy of welfare organized through NGOs. . . . They are imagined as places where people learn . . . to organize their bodies and lives in terms of the requirements of antiretroviral therapy" (Prince 2012: 109). However, there were no support groups in Tari. In short, there was little in the Tari context to suggest that the clinic exerted significant power to produce compliant patient-subjects.

Most of the women I interviewed were, nevertheless, highly compliant with most of the recommended behaviors (the men I interviewed were not). Thus, my point here is not that HIV clinical care in Papua New Guinea does not exert governmental and disciplinary effects, but rather that in analyzing how patient compliance is produced, it is important to consider not only clinical discourses and practices, but also how these intersect with context-specific, gendered expectations and patients' lived experiences in their families and communities. A theoretical framework that overemphasizes the power of the clinic risks obfuscating the role of a patient's family and social networks, or the lack of them (see also Meinert et al. 2009). For example, some of the women I interviewed were profoundly lonely, having been cut off by family and sometimes friends. "I don't have any besties," Shelly said. "My only friends really are the nurses here. I have one friend who is also HIV-positive that I met here at the clinic, but we live too far away from each other. I only see her when we come pick up our medicine at the same time." In this state of solitary abandon, women like Shelly worked to insert themselves into the life of the clinic and to befriend the health workers, often bringing them small gifts (betel nut, a roasted sweet potato). So, while the clinics in Tari did not seem to exert much disciplinary force, being compliant to "the rules of ART" was sometimes framed by patients as an act of deference that they hoped would help build a relationship of care between themselves and the health workers. In other words, the governmental relationship may result not only from clinical disciplinary acts, but also from the accretion of patients' gestures of submission and their overtures of intimacy that gradually entwine their subjectivities with clinical expectations.

This will to comply is also reinforced by gendered expectations of comportment. In general, Huli women' s reputations—that is, their moral capital—benefit from being seen to comply with rules and expectations. Women are praised when they are known to regularly attend church, work in their sweet potato fields, obey their husband's rules (e.g., asking permission to visit natal kin or not touching a husband's belongings), and put others' needs and desires before their own. Thus, many women expressed pride about their rigorous medication adherence. Families also pressure patients to be compliant, in part for their health, of course, but also as a demonstration of their willingness to be "fenced in" by the "laws" of ART. Thus, women are motivated to be compliant in part because of clinicians' governmental exertions and in part to demonstrate to family their moral intentions (a topic discussed at more length in the next chapter).

AIDS AS AN AFFECTIVE DISORDER

The other directive that health workers typically gave HIV-positive patients was that they should try not to worry and should avoid other negative emotions, such as anger. Rasmussen similarly lists "maintaining a positive attitude" as one of the "rules" that patients in Uganda are told to follow. The enjoinder to "live positively" can be traced to the early days of the epidemic in North America, a time of powerful stigma and no treatment (Dilger 2001, Hardon 2012). "Positive living" is wordplay that urges the HIV-positive to come to terms with their sero-status, to maintain an optimistic outlook, and to care for themselves both physically and emotionally (Levy and Storeng 2007, Benton et al. 2017). The wordplay does not work particularly well in Tari, where many patients are not fluent in English, but the intent of the directive—to have hope and to avoid pessimism and despair—remains, and has been translated into the advice not to worry and to avoid negative feelings. Anger and worry, patients are told, can "wake up the virus" (which has been put to sleep by ARVs) or cause their medications to be less effective. Importantly, this advice enters a cultural context that has specific philosophies about emotion, especially anger, and where ethnic identity is strongly tied to a specific affective style.

Avoiding Anger

Huli associate themselves as a group with a very specific emotional style: the ability to move rapidly from one emotional state to another, and especially from anger to cheerfulness. "The most important thing to understand about us is that our emotions fluctuate," a Huli university student told me. To outsiders, this fluctuation or volatility—in which a person can be in a rage one minute and laughing a minute or two later—can be disconcerting and even a little frightening. I have had many conversations with Papua New Guineans recently moved to Tari, or with Peace Corps or MSF volunteers, about their unnerving interactions with Huli people who were shaking with rage and threatening violence, and a short time later were sheepishly mocking themselves for their outburst. This emotional style may look like volatility, but volatility connotes lack of control, and Huli assert that their affective ideal requires a great deal of control, making it something more like affective suppleness or agility. Edward Schieffelin, writing about the Kaluli, a neighboring group, observes:

> A man's temper, or 'tendency to get angry,' is an important feature by which Kaluli judge his character and assess the degree to which he is a force to be reckoned with. It represents the vigor with which he will stand up for or pursue his interest vis-à-vis others, and the likelihood that he will retaliate for wrong or injury. . . . When Kaluli feel strongly about something, they are not usually ones to hide their feelings. Rage, grief, dismay, embarrassment, fear, and compassion may be openly and often dramatically expressed. . . . These displays of affect have to be seen more as declarations of mind, motivation, and/or intention than as mere cathartic expressions of feeling. (Schieffelin 1983: 183–84)

This passage describes the Huli equally well, though their self-representations emphasize also their capacity for joy and jocularity, as much as their capacity for rage. And, the ability to move nimbly between these expressive states is as important as successfully performing the states themselves.

Huli readily acknowledge that not every Huli person can master this affective suppleness. Women, in particular, are often said to be incapable of this ideal, because they are "unable to let go of anger." Arguably, Huli women have much to be angry about, whether it is domestic violence, denigrating discourses about female inferiority, male sexual privilege, polygyny, or an unfair burden of domestic labor. Nevertheless, many Huli women also assert that affective suppleness is a distinctive Huli cultural characteristic, and an ideal to strive for, and that women are less able to achieve it because of their tendency to feel lingering rancor.

Commenting on the relationship between feminist theory and affect theory, Carolyn Pedwell and Anne Whitehead note that feminist scholars have long pointed out the "critical links between affect and gendered . . . relations of power" (Pedwell and Whitehead 2012: 116). For example, a woman's display of emotion can be used to suggest her lack of rationality and thus to delegitimize and dismiss her point of view (Ahmed 2010, Jaggar 1989, Lutz 1995). Or, women's fitness for positions of political and economic power have been questioned because of their supposed emotional instability due to hormonal cycles. Or, women's presumed innate tender feelings have been used to argue that their proper place is in the home. In short, discourse about affect is often a kind of ideological material for cementing gendered hierarchies. In this case, Huli women's alleged tendencies to be less emotionally nimble than men—and, in particular, to experience stubborn, persistent anger—are decontextualized from the situations and relations of inequality that produce them and are naturalized as an innately female affective deficiency, a quality that makes them "less Huli" than Huli men.

Alongside this ideal of affective nimbleness is an equally strong model that emphasizes the physiological danger of suppressing anger and the importance of expressing it. Huli women describe anger quite viscerally as a powerful and hot sensation that begins in the belly, rises up through the throat, often impeding speech and breathing, and enters the head, causing an intense pressure that can effect vision, hearing, and the ability to think. Anger bottled up causes illness. Theresa, for example, attributed her elderly father's dementia to his habit of keeping his anger bottled up inside:

> He's always been a man who talks very little, especially when he's angry. He'll only make his argument once, and then if he feels that he's not being heard he won't talk about it anymore. He doesn't let his anger out. And this has made him sick many times. And now that he's old, it has made him senile (*longlong*).

As one might imagine, these ideas about anger—the feminization of enduring anger, the danger of unexpressed anger—create a conundrum for HIV-positive women when they are told to avoid it: if they experience anger, they might have a hard time letting go of it, and if they bottle it up, they may aggravate their symptoms. Avoiding anger is also problematic because anger is often valued by Huli women as an agency-enhancing emotion—it gives one the energy to respond to other people's affronts. Responding with verbal and physical aggression to violations—such as others stealing from you or hitting you—is actively socialized in boys and girls and considered appropriate behavior for both men and women. Thus, while women are lauded for abiding by gendered expectations, including obedience, this should not be taken to mean that they are rewarded for being passive or docile. Most of the women I've interviewed over the years have spoken proudly of the physical fights they've been in, and women who do not attempt to punish transgressors may be viewed as cowards who are easily victimized. All of the HIV-positive women I interviewed, however, described trying to "fence in," "lose," or "forget" their anger, which meant walking away from others' transgressions, a deeply conflicted struggle for many of them.

Martha's story of how she came to be tested for HIV, and her efforts to control her emotions post-diagnosis, illustrates how "fencing in one's anger" poses a challenge. Martha's husband, a civil servant, had been transferred to another highlands town, leaving Martha and their four children in Tari. He had eventually taken a second wife without telling Martha, and upon learning about the marriage from other people, she traveled to this town with the specific aim of beating up the new wife:

> I had gone to Mendi because I wanted to beat up my husband's second wife, a Pangia woman. And while we were fighting she said, "I have AIDS and I've given it to your husband, so you better watch out!" [She just said it straight out like that?] Yes, she said it just like that. We were yelling and fighting, and so she said it like that to shock me. She wanted to win the fight, and she hoped that if I were shocked my body would suddenly become weak. And she was right. I was terrified, and my body

lost all its strength, and I lost the fight. Then I went and got a blood test, and it was positive. . . . [How did your family respond when they found out?] They felt sorry for me. They said, "You are a good woman who just stays at home, and you never act like the wife of a civil servant. This was your husband's fault—you didn't do this, he did this. But don't worry, you'll be fine." . . . [How have you been about taking your medicine? Have you had any problems?] At first I hated taking the medicine—every pill I took reminded me that I had HIV and that my husband had infected me. I was worried and angry all the time, every time I swallowed a pill, and so the medicine didn't work very well. My skin turned dark black and my eyes turned yellow. But finally I stopped being so angry, and now the medicine works well. . . . [And do you get along with your husband now? Can you talk to him or do you get angry with him for infecting you?] I stop myself from getting angry with him. If I get angry, my body gets worse. My skin turns dark and dusty. It is the worry and anger that does it. So I've given up anger and worry. I've schooled myself to give up these feelings. [How do you do that?] When I feel myself getting angry I try to quickly think about something else, or I walk away from the situation. And I tell myself over and over that I need to be afraid of getting angry. Normal people may get angry, but we people with this sickness may not get angry.

Here Martha draws a direct connection between her family's assessment of her moral character and how they responded to her being HIV-positive. Her character is sound because she was sexually faithful ("you are a good woman who just stays at home") and because she has never "acted like the wife of a civil servant" (that is, as if she is superior to others); thus, her family was willing to take her in when she left her husband. Also important is the distinction that she draws between "normal" people and HIV-positive people: normal people can feel anger without considering the health consequences, whereas the HIV-positive need to "school" themselves not to feel it. Thus, Martha self-monitors and disciplines her anger, and even deliberately mobilizes another emotion—fear (that is, the fear of her ARVs failing and of dying)—to control her anger.

Feminist scholars' engagements with affect theory are useful here for thinking about the implications and consequences of the instruction to avoid anger. Scholars like Erin Rand have emphasized "the epistemological function of affect and emotion in public discourse" (Rand 2015: 173)—that is, the way that authoritative directives to *feel* a particular way about an experience both shape what we are able to *know* about it and work to foreclose other ways of knowing. For example, Sara Ahmed argues that the cultural imperative to be happy about heteronormative ideals works to silence critical questions about those ideals (Ahmed 2010; see also Cvetkovich 2012). In the case of HIV-positive women, the instruction to avoid anger has both disciplinary and epistemological effects: it shapes both how women behave and how they know and experience their condition of being HIV-positive. For one thing, this directive guides them to think of their emotions as internal, privately owned feeling states whose most vital connections are to their own individual immune systems and viral loads. In other words, it directs them to look inward towards assiduous self-monitoring, rather than outward towards shared experience. As such, it reinforces the idea that women should *know* their HIV-positive status as an individual, rather than a social, condition.

Furthermore, because this directive frames anger as an individual health concern—pathologizes it, in a sense—it occludes the possibility of experiencing anger as a shared sociopolitical diagnostic or impetus to action. Feminist scholars have long pointed out that emotions, rather than being idiosyncratic, nonrational sensations, can be seen as somatic indices of inequality or as "indications that something is wrong with the way alleged facts have been constructed, with accepted understandings of how things are. . . . Only when we reflect on our initially puzzling irritability, revulsion, anger or fear may we bring to consciousness our 'gut-level' awareness that we are in a situation of coercion, cruelty, injustice or danger" (Jaggar 1989: 167). More recently, Geraldine Pratt and Victoria Rosner have observed that, "For many feminists emotion can be a potent analytic tool for discerning social injustices. . . . In this context anger has been of special importance" (Pratt and Rosner 2012: 5). Telling HIV-positive women to "fence in" their emotions, eschew anger, and to walk away from situations that cause upset is thus telling them to give up an important epistemological tool for seeing the structures of inequality that have made them vulnerable to infection. Indeed, some, like Zoli, come to distrust and denigrate their own feelings of anger.

Zoli had a 6th grade education and was in her mid forties when I met her. She had a daughter who was also HIV-positive, likely infected by her policeman husband. When young, Zoli had married a Huli man and moved to Mt. Hagen, where he worked. Over time they had five children together, and because his employer provided housing, they were able to save money to buy a small house and rent it out. She recalled:

> But then he made a lot of money from renting out this house, and his salary increased, and so he married another wife. He didn't think about me, and he didn't give me money. He didn't give me money for the children. He just dropped us, and he didn't take care of us anymore. And he kicked us out of the company house, so he could live there with his new wife, and he sent us home to Tari. . . . [So when he did this, what happened? I think you must have been angry.] Yes, I was very angry. I passengered around. I wanted to show him that if he wanted to go around, I could go around too (*em laik raun, mi tu bai raun*). I passengered around in Mt. Hagen. I left my children and went to Port Moresby and passengered around. And finally I came back to Tari and lived with my mother. But then she died. And I went crazy. My thinking became confused (*tingting bilong mi faul*). My husband left me, my mother who took care of me died—my thinking completely crashed (*tingting bilong mi krash olgeta*). So I left my children again and went to Madang. I passengered around in Madang. Then I met a Huli man there who said he would take care of me. And I thought it was a good idea—he could help me take care of my children. But it turned out he was sick. That's how I got this sickness.

When I asked how she was sure it was this man in Madang who had infected her, given her many other sexual partners, she replied, "It's true I had sex with a lot of men—in Mt. Hagen, in Port Moresby, in Madang. But I used condoms. The only reason I didn't use a condom with the man in Madang is because I thought we were going to get married"—an explanation that echoes a wealth of research demonstrating that women often use condoms with transactional sexual partners or customers, but that more intimate, trusting, longer-term relationships are marked as such through foregoing condoms (Varga 1997, Tavory and Swidler 2009).

When her family found out about her HIV-positive status, "They said I had brought this problem on myself. And it's true that I left Tari in anger, and then I crashed. That's how I damaged myself (*mi kros wantaim na mi go, na mi krash nau. Olsem na mi bagarapim mi yet*)." Here, Zoli ruefully suggests that her family was not wrong in their judgment of her: her own anger, she said, was responsible for her HIV-positive status. It was anger about her husband's behavior that drove her to act in the sexually reckless manner that ultimately resulted in infection. I reminded her that by her own account she had been infected when she was attempting to behave as a "good" woman, trying to forge a new marriage. However, the fact that she now considered anger to be a "bad" and unhealthy feeling that could worsen her HIV-positive condition led her to conclude that anger was also responsible for her infection in the first place. In other words, her new understanding of anger led to a rethinking and negative reevaluation of the role it had played in her past.

Feminist scholars have debated not only the epistemological role of emotion in how we come to know our own experiences, but its role in political life, asking whether the labile, unpredictable, multiplicitous nature of affect enriches our understandings of humans as political subjects, and indicates that subjectification/subjection is never total, or whether, in contrast, affect is a powerful means through which domination is exercised, through, for example, attaching subjects to nationalist or to racial ideologies (Sedgwick 2003, Ahmed 2010, Koivunen 2010, Bargetz 2015). Influenced by Spinoza, and his conceptualization of affect as a force that can increase or decrease our capacity to act, scholars have debated the nature of specific emotions for agency. Rosi Braidotti argues, for example, that feminist political action should be grounded in "an ethics of joy and affirmation" (Braidotti 2002: 13). Sara Ahmed, in contrast, asserts that anger is key to political mobilization: "Crucially anger is not simply defined in relationship to a past, but as opening up the future. . . . As [Audre] Lorde shows us, anger is visionary, and the fear of anger, or the transformation of anger into silence, is a turning away from the future" (Ahmed [2004] 2015: 175). Ahmed cites Lorde's analysis of her own anger about racism: "Anger expressed and translated into action in the service of our vision and our future is a liberating and strengthening act of clarification . . . Anger is loaded with information and energy" (Lorde 1984: 124, 127). And, in her

138 CARING FOR THE SELF

2010 book *The Promise of Happiness*, Ahmed posits the feminist "killjoy" as a marginalized but crucial political voice whose anger is necessary for identifying oppressive social structures and galvanizing action against them (Ahmed 2010: 20).

Reading the HIV clinic's admonition to avoid anger in light of this theorizing suggests that it has both governmental and anti-political effects. It not only translates anger into a health condition that requires monitoring of one's interior self, it also encourages women to fear it. Fully experiencing anger about HIV stigma, for example, might generate shared narratives about living with HIV, which might in turn pave the way for other affective possibilities, such as fellow feelings of solidarity, hope, or determined resolve (Berlant 2011). The taboo against anger arguably turns women away from this future. I should be clear that I do not think that this is the intent of health workers. On the contrary, their intent is both to help patients live longer and to enhance the quality of patients' lives by giving them permission to remove themselves from the affective rough-and-tumble of everyday life in Tari. They know that patients can be objects of fear and suspicion, and one of their aims is to give patients a good reason *not* to respond to others' aggressions.

AIDS and Worry

Although HIV-positive women considered anger dangerous to their health, the emotion most associated with HIV/AIDS in Tari was worry. Indeed, a dominant model of AIDS before the arrival of antiretrovirals was that it was worrying that killed infected people, not the virus (Andersen 2017, Hinton and Earnest 2010). Some of the evangelical churches in Tari promoted this construction of HIV/AIDS and asserted that being "born again" was the only solution to fatal worrying: putting one's faith in God and trusting in his divine, if unknowable, plan allowed one to lay down one's worries. With the arrival of ARVs in 2007, this model lost most of its purchase, since patients were seen to recover their health without being born again. Nevertheless, the ruinous effects of worry remained a compelling concern for patients.

When I asked clinic staff about this concern, they said that patients used two Huli words to talk about their worries: *genda,* which refers to a feeling of heaviness, and *mini purugu,* which refers to thinking compulsively about a situation. Patients and clinicians alike described both kinds as lodging inside the body and causing physical damage. Patients worried about a range of things: being abandoned, dying and leaving their children with no one to care for them, being hated by spouses and children for "bringing AIDS into the family" (a worry expressed more by men), having land stolen by avaricious and scheming kin, and, for those without children, leaving no lineal trace of themselves into the future. A very common worry was malicious gossip, which one patient described to me as "when you know that people are spreading rumors about you, and especially saying ugly things about your sick body, or about how you will die soon, or about the bad things you must have done to get HIV."

The patients I interviewed often spoke in great detail about the worries they tried not to have: "You imagine your family and friends living on without you. For example, you will all be around a fire talking, and then suddenly you'll imagine the same scene, but you are missing, erased from the picture. And you try to go to sleep, but now you can't stop picturing this." Here, the person living with HIV experiences a moment of reflection that removes her from being in the moment and forces her to imagine a typical family tableau in the future, without her. And once she has imagined this, she finds it difficult not to imagine other family and community gatherings in the same way. Another elaborately detailed worry that a few women described themselves as trying not to experience was:

> You compare yourself with friends who don't have HIV. For example, you see some-one you grew up with, and before you were on the same life path. And then she went to school and you didn't, or you had to drop out because no money. And now she has *more* money, she has a family, she is thriving, and you feel that you have lost all of those things, or never had those things. If you had money, it is now gone, and no one will give you anything.

This is an affectively dense and layered form of worry that combines loss, envy, anger, and despair. It sums up life circumstances that can put one on a path to HIV infection, as well as what can happen afterwards. It also constitutes a kind of rebuttal to the still dominant public health model of HIV causality, which focuses on individual risk behaviors rather than the intersecting inequalities that propel behavior or put one in the path of someone else's behavior. It might also be seen as one of Pratt's and Rosner's (2012) affective analytic tools for discerning social injustices: it is a distressing feeling that causes its experiencer to reflect on how dif-ferent life circumstances—for example, having the funds to attend school or not—can lead to stark differential outcomes, such as being infected with HIV, which, in turn, can lead to a cascade of social and material losses. However, worry does not afford as much potential for action as anger does.

We might therefore think of "worry" in this context as similar to one of Sianne Ngai's "ugly feelings"—that is, feelings that are "minor and generally unprestigious . . . *non*cathartic, offering no satisfactions of virtue . . . nor any therapeutic or puri-fying release" (Ngai 2005: 6, emphasis in original). Much like the affect theorists discussed above, Ngai is influenced by Spinoza's conceptualization of emotions as "'waverings of the mind' that can either increase or diminish one's power to act"—that is, she grapples with the relationships between affect and agency (2). However, rather than focus on the noble feeling-scapes typically analyzed by literary schol-ars, such as tragedy, Ngai instead mines films and novels for scenes character-ized by affects that are "experientially negative, in the sense that they evoke pain or displeasure," as well as "semantically negative, in the sense that they are satu-rated with socially stigmatizing meanings and values" (11). Such scenes, she says, often convey "ambivalent situations of suspended agency" (1). In other words, ugly feelings obstruct a protagonist's ability to act, move forward, or be transformed. For Ngai these include envy, irritation, and anxiety. Worry was similarly described by women living with HIV as a paralyzing feeling that could impede their ability to care for themselves and others.

EMOTIONAL REGULATION AS A PRACTICE
OF SELF-CARE

As suggested by the narratives of Martha, Zoli, and Shelly, the women I interviewed took to heart the injunction not to worry or get angry, and they had developed a range of strategies for managing negative feelings. Some of these were aimed at modulating one's interior emotional life, and some were aimed more externally at limiting one's exposure to people and situations that might cause upset. I separate these into four categories: religious faith, emotional diversion, social avoidance, and rejecting remarriage.

Religious Faith

In the face of hostility from kin, a determined faith that they had a place in God's unknowable plan was sometimes the only thing that enabled women to leave the house and persevere. Over the course of my three years doing these interviews, I myself was sometimes used to illustrate the rightness of refusing worry and having faith in God: at the end of an interview, when compensating interviewees for participating in the research, a few woman said something along the lines of, "You see? I came to pick up my medication this morning, knowing that I did not have money to buy food in town or even for the PMV fare home, but I refused to worry because I know God will take care of me. And then you were here, and we talked, and you gave me money."

Faith that God would provide not only gave them emotional comfort, but also the bravery to take risks, such as hopping on a PMV without knowing if they would be able to get home at the end of the day, a finding that reinforces the importance of examining faith not only as a cognitive matter of "belief," but also as an affectively rich state of mind that provides far more than solace. Although some ethnographic research suggests that heightened religious zeal may motivate patients to abandon their ARVs in the faith that God can heal them (Burchardt 2014), the small acts of courageous faith by the women I interviewed were often for the sake of self-care: to get the next three months supply of ARVs, no matter what, or to find food and company.

Emotional Diversion

Diverting oneself to drive worries from one's mind was also a common strategy. A few women, for example, spoke of going regularly to Tari's large main market in hope of running into friends and family who might engross them in banter or news about disputes and village court cases. Arguably, they were lonely and seeking out company and social interaction, and yet they often framed this as a quest to divert themselves from negative thoughts that might otherwise preoccupy them. If they stayed at home, they said, there would be nothing to prevent them from dwelling on their worries, but at the Tari market they were likely to run into people who would take a moment to share gossip or make them laugh. Family members also sometimes helped with this strategy of emotional diversion: some women's sisters, for example, said they would send their young children to entertain them because "children say and do funny things that make grown-ups laugh, and we don't want her to worry."

What might be called cell phone sociality also had a very important role to play in this strategy of emotional diversion. Almost all of the women who owned mobile phones had long lists of "phone friends." The "phone friend" phenomenon has been described as "a uniquely PNG response to the communicative possibilities of the mobile phone" (Andersen 2013: 319). It is the calling of, or accepting a call from, unknown phone numbers with the aim of forming a friendship or romance with a stranger that will likely exist only by phone and may endure for one phone call or for many months. Most people I knew in Tari had phone friends, and many of these were romantic partners who would flirt, confide woes, offer sympathy, and sometimes send each other phone credit. The HIV-positive women I interviewed had both male and female phone friends, and while some of these connections were romantic or flirtatious in nature, most women said that they spoke to these friends late at night if they had a sudden attack of worry. When they found themselves *tingting plenti* (thinking a lot), *wari wari* (worrying a lot), or *busy tumas* (very busy, but it can also mean overly preoccupied with or perseverating about something), they would call their phone friends, who could calm or distract them with teasing, chatty, or comforting talk.

Phone friends were, in effect, affective regulators, helping the women to modulate their anxious thoughts and emotions (Wardlow 2018). They were especially important for women like Last Minute Lucy, who had been shunned by natal kin and were living alone. Indeed, when I spoke with Lucy a year after I first interviewed her, her phone had just been stolen and she was distraught. Because she had not actually met any of her phone friends face-to-face, had not memorized their numbers, and had no other way of contacting them, they were all lost to her. "My thoughts (*tingting bilong mi*) are fucked up," she said over and over. "All those phone friends, in Port Moresby and other places. They would send me credit, and we talked all the time, every night, and now I don't have a phone and I've lost all those numbers. My thoughts are fucked up."

Social Avoidance

The strategies described above are specifically aimed at preventing worry, not anger, which for some women was a more difficult emotion to manage, because its instigation was less under their control. Whereas worry was usually triggered by their own thoughts about a situation, anger was more often triggered by interaction with others. For women who had been rejected by their families, it was running into them and enduring their slights, insults, or refusals to help that caused anger. Like Martha, some "schooled" themselves to walk away from inflammatory encounters, not easy in a context where, as noted above, summoning up a splendid rage and standing up for oneself verbally and physically are highly valued.

Others, wanting to avoid the possibility of anger altogether, cut themselves off from important social spaces. Much Huli socializing takes place, not in people's homes, but more publicly, whether on the road or on church premises or in the marketplace or a community area for playing sport and hearing village court cases. Some women said that they took great care in trying to avoid many of these spaces because they never knew whom they might see there: an unexpected run-in with a past nemesis, a husband's other wife, or relatives who had cast one out might result in an argument or altercation, which could negatively impact one's health.

Rosina, for example, said she now avoided going to weekly women's basketball games because of an incident in which she had been shamed in public. As she described it, there had been a dispute about the game she was participating in, and women from both teams, including herself, had begun insulting each other. Then a woman from the other team, who had recently divorced Rosina's brother and knew she was HIV-positive, pointed at her and yelled, "the AIDS germs inside her are making her say all kinds of things. Let's just drop it and leave—AIDS has made her crazy." She found herself yelling back,

> Those germs aren't making me do anything. I didn't go out and find these germs; my husband gave them to me. And why are you talking about my germs in public?! Do you think you can shock people here and shame me? Everyone here knows. I have not hidden this—I have told everyone in my community about this. So why are you trying to shame me in public?

The insults back and forth escalated, and then the yelling turned into a physical fight between the two families, with other people joining in. In the end, the woman had to give Rosina K200 for "calling me an AIDS woman in public."

Notice that Rosina makes a point of establishing her own unblemished moral character: she asserts that she herself did not "find" HIV—that is, her infection was not due to her own illicit sexual behavior; rather, she was an innocent party, infected by her husband. She also asserts that lest the insulter believe that she is conveying some shocking revelation by announcing Rosina's HIV status to everyone at the basketball game, in fact Rosina has made a point of disclosing her status to her whole community, an issue I expand upon in the next chapter in connection with the ethical challenges and imperatives of living with HIV in Tari. Since the national HAMP (HIV/AIDS Management and Prevention) Act of 2003 makes it unlawful to stigmatize a person because they are infected or affected by HIV/AIDS, and because Huli custom allows people to demand compensation from those who publicly insult them, the insulter's family had to give Rosina compensation.

Although Rosina was vindicated by this experience, she felt she could not risk that kind of altercation again. So she stopped participating in, or even attending, community basketball games. This was in part because she did not want to embroil her family in any more conflicts regarding her HIV status, but it was also because she was afraid of the anger she had experienced. She acknowledged that getting angry during this basketball game, and feeling her family get angry with and for her, was, in fact, a pleasurable experience, but she worried that any similar affective assaults on her immune system might make her ill. In short, the effort to prevent anger can lead HIV-positive women to remove themselves from the daily fabric of social life.

It is also worth noting that in forsaking anger, HIV-positive women are not only forsaking valued, and even relished, modes of social interaction, but also sometimes justice. Last Minute Lucy, for example, said that she had been raising nine chickens, but a neighbor's dog killed a few and some "marijuana faces" (young men who are known to smoke pot) stole the rest. "They weren't outsiders," Lucy said.

> They were from my community. I think they thought that an HIV-positive woman doesn't deserve to be successful raising and selling chickens, and that I wouldn't be able to do anything about it. I wanted to take all these people to village court and demand compensation. But I dropped it. I don't want to get angry, and if I take them to court, they will lie and insult me and make me angry. So I dropped it.

Village court cases can be unruly public events, where tempers are lost, lies unleashed, and insults exchanged. Anticipating that her feelings would be riled by the denials and slurs of the people she accused, Lucy decided not to go forward at all. Similarly, Shelly—who, as noted above, was homeless and sometimes slept under a mosquito net in people's sweet potato fields—said this about how she responded when her family evicted her:

> They kicked me out and they harvested what I had planted. [And did this make you angry?] Yes, but I could feel the anger making my sickness worse. If I worry and get angry, then my body will lose weight. So I had to let go of my anger. I must fence myself in (*banisim mi yet*) so that I don't get angry and I don't worry (*mi noken kros, noken wari*). . . . So, you want to steal my food, fine. I'll just leave.

Zoli too said that she and her HIV-positive daughter had been evicted from her father's land:

> They wouldn't let us stay. They took everything—the blankets, the mattresses, our land, our house. They broke the walls, tore down the house, stole everything. So now we live on my mother's land with my sister. . . . I work hard—I wash all the plates

and wash all the clothes. But sometimes they are unhappy with me. I try to humble myself (*mi trai na hamblim mi yet*) and work hard and not worry. . . . Problems come, but I try not to worry. If I worry too much, I might die. Sometimes I find myself thinking, "I haven't seen my daughter in a while—I'm worried about her" or "My brother hit me" or "My sister's husband is mad at me and might kick me out." But I try not to think about these things. If I think about it too much, I am killing myself.

In short, avoiding anger sometimes meant letting others infringe upon one with impunity or humbling oneself and hoping for others' tolerance.

Rejecting Remarriage

Thirteen of the women I interviewed were widows and ten were divorced, and almost all of these women had received one or more marriage proposals since being diagnosed HIV-positive, typically from men who didn't know them, but who had learned that they were available (in the sense that all widows and divorced women are considered available). All but one of the women rejected these proposals by informing the men of their HIV status and asserting that they didn't want to risk infecting them. In other words, they let the men believe that it was only their HIV status that prevented them from accepting the proposal. However, when I asked whether they wanted to remarry, most of them replied with an adamant no. This was my exchange with Gloria:

> I don't have worries and I'm not afraid. If got married again I would start worrying again—I would worry about food and about money. But the way I live now I have my two hands and I can take care of myself and not worry. . . . I want to be faithful to the medicine. (Here, Gloria was deliberately playing on the command to "Be faithful" from ABC prevention messages: being faithful to her husband had not prevented her from being infected with HIV, but being faithful to her medication kept her alive and happy.) [What have the nurses told you about remarrying?] They have said that I can. But. But. I don't want to (*mi les*). . . . Here—Highlands men, they are no good. If you have a little money, they'll say, "I'll boss it," and then they'll just take it—they'll go into your string bag and just take it. That's how they are. I was already married, and I know what it's like. We physically fought all the time, and he slept with lots of women, and caused me a lot of worry. And now I'm not married and I'm happier than ever. I'm relaxed. So, why should I go around and look for another husband? I'm not interested.

Lucy, for her part, used concerns about excess worry to leave her second husband:

> Even after we tested positive he continued to passenger around and get drunk with his friends and go to *dawe anda*. I tried to control him, but I couldn't. I told him he needed to stay at home, eat better food, get enough sleep, and wash every day, and he just wouldn't. And I was worried he might infect someone else and there might be "trouble." (Recall that "trouble" is a euphemism for compensation demands, retaliatory violence, or tribal fighting.) It was causing me too much worry and pressure, and I felt myself getting worse because I was worrying about him and his behavior.

I told him, "We are patients. That means we are a different kind of person now. We have to behave differently." But he wouldn't listen. So finally I explained that he was causing me too much worry and that it would be better if we lived apart. So we divided up everything fairly—the chickens, the pigs, the bedding, the pots and pans, the clothes. And then I left. I told him to call me when he got really sick. I said I would come see him. And he did get really sick, and a nurse called me, and I came. He said, "I am dying, and you are still alive. But that's okay." And then he died.

When I asked if she wanted to remarry, Lucy replied:

I have seen my own marriages and other people's marriages, and I have seen how men behave when they marry you, and really I hate them (*mi save hetim ol*). They control you—tell you you can't go to the market or that you have to cook something for them. And then they are quick to get cross or hit you if you disobey. So really I hate them. I've had HIV-positive men ask me if I will marry them, but I think married life is no good. It just causes anger and fights and worry. If I thought a man would care for me and not get angry, then maybe. But I haven't seen any men like that.

Many women suggested that one had to choose between marriage and a healthy life. The one benefit of HIV stigma, such as it was, was that many people viewed the HIV-positive as unmarriageable. Showing men their ARVs or clinic books was therefore an expedient way for women to deftly decline proposals. Thus, while public health practitioners have sometimes conceptualized marriage as a state that can protect people from HIV, the women I interviewed saw their HIV-positivity as a state that protected them from marriage.

Their desires to avoid marriage contrast markedly with findings elsewhere. Kathryn Rhine, for example, found that HIV-positive women in Nigeria wanted to marry and have children; they participated in AIDS support groups largely to find potential mates (Rhine 2009). This difference speaks, I think, to the strife-ridden nature of many Huli marriages. However, it is also important to bear in mind that, compared with Rhine's interlocutors, the women I interviewed were, on average, much older and already had children. They had thus already fulfilled their womanly obligations to bring in bridewealth for their natal families and bear children for their husbands' families. Had my sample been younger, I believe more women might have expressed a desire to marry.

CONCLUSION

The advice to avoid negative emotions was a health message that most of the women I interviewed took to heart, more even than instructions about nutrition or stopping smoking. Being attentive to their feelings and trying to regulate them became an important form of self-care, and many spoke of AIDS almost as an affective disorder, in the sense that one's emotions could play an outsized role in whether the virus remained "asleep," or "fenced in," or "woke up" and "broke out of the fence." This construction of AIDS resonates with Marian Burchardt's find-ings in South Africa, in which "infection emerges as a psychological disease, as an affliction that impairs life by constantly reminding the infected person of possible future suffering" (Burchardt 2014: 63). In both cases it is the affective dimensions of being HIV-positive that are sometimes experienced as so corrosive that they can cause biological death. And the women I interviewed often read their own bodily signs, such as skin ulcers and fevers, as indications that their emotions had gotten the better of them.

Some women were more concerned about anger because they felt less able to control the external circumstances that could incite it. They anticipated, for exam-ple, that if someone insulted them on the road, not only would they feel anger about the insult, but this anger would also be intensified by the humiliation they experienced when they forced themselves to walk away without responding. Not all women were successful at walking away from others' emotional assaults, of course, or even tried very hard in some cases. Peony, for example, had been living with her husband in 2012, when I first interviewed her, but wasn't in 2013; between the two interviews, her husband, who had infected her, abandoned her and mar-ried another HIV-positive woman he had met at the clinic. Smiling somewhat sheepishly, she said she began working on not feeling anger *after* she burned down his house. More women were concerned about worry, however. And although some women described elaborate worry scenarios—such as imagining themselves as entirely absent from future family gatherings, or imagining their orphaned children at the mercy of neglectful or abusive kin—others did not even want to talk about their worries, for fear that talking about them would bring them to mind. "I don't worry," a couple of women said, abruptly putting an end to that line of inquiry.

Worry can be seen as one of Ngai's "ugly feelings"—dysphoric emotions that suspend agency. The bodily heaviness of worry, or compulsive thinking about problems, paralyzed some women. In these cases, the clinical advice to try not to worry did seem to help them, and indeed motivated some of them to seek out company, talk, gossip, and laughter. For others, it motivated a redoubling of religious faith, which they found consoling, and sometimes even revitalizing.

The advice to avoid anger, on the other hand, often posed some problems. Recall Edward Schieffelin's observation about the neighboring Kaluli that emo-tions such as anger "may be openly and often dramatically expressed. . . . These displays of affect have to be seen more as declarations of mind, motivation, and/or intention than as mere cathartic expressions of feeling" (Schieffelin 1983: 183–84). In other words, a display of anger is often an assertion about oneself—that one is not the kind of person to tolerate others' insults or offences, and that one intends to take serious action should the offense continue. The performance of anger can thus be important for maintaining others' respect and one's own sense of dignity, and among the Huli, this is true of women as well as of men. Moreover, as noted by feminist scholars of affect and by Huli women, anger can enhance one's sense of agency. As Audre Lorde put it, anger can be a "strengthening act of clarification. . . . Anger is loaded with information and energy" (Lorde 1984: 124, 127).

In some cases, the advice to avoid anger led to a kind of self-exclusion in the name of caring for the self, with women withdrawing from social venues and activities with the aim of protecting themselves from potential upset. As important, the directive to avoid negative emotions often motivated a turning inward of attention, and it fostered an understanding of emotions as private feeling states connected to one's own personal bodily condition, rather than as shared responses to experiences held in common. In other words, it furthered an individualization of the experience of being HIV-positive. This individualization, along with the lack of support groups in Tari, meant that there was little sense of collective experience, let alone solidarity, between women living with HIV.

6

"Like Normal"

The Ethics of Living with HIV

Recall Kelapi from chapter 1. In return for being allowed to live on his land, and a cash payment of K700, Kelapi's aunt and uncle, Huli migrants in Porgera, facilitated her rape and abduction by a neighboring landowner, who then took her as an additional wife.[1] After she tested HIV-positive and fled home to Tari, she was one of the first patients to seek help at the Catholic AIDS Care Centre:

> I was the second person here when the AIDS Care Centre opened. A lot of people were too afraid to come, and at that time there were no ARVs, only (the antibiotic) Bactrim. . . . [So when you ran away and came back home, did you tell your family that you had this sickness?] Yes, I told them, but think, at this time everyone was terrified of AIDS. It was still new and there was no medicine, so everyone was afraid. My family wouldn't touch me, they didn't want to hand things to me, they didn't want me to eat with them. I was very thin, like a bony, bony chicken, but they didn't want to share food with me.

When ARVs became available at the Care Centre in 2007, Kelapi thrived, and eventually she was well enough to become a volunteer at a small elementary school.[2] She was one of the few HIV-positive women I interviewed who wanted to remarry and did so. She fell in love with a good friend of mine, a kind and thoughtful Huli man I'd known since my doctoral fieldwork, although she and I didn't realize this connection between us until after the interview.

> I went to this little bush school to teach elementary (students) and I met him, and he didn't think I had AIDS. We worked together, and when he looked at me he thought I was a healthy, normal woman, and he wanted to marry me. And I was honest with him, "My body may look healthy, but I'm taking AIDS medicine. You shouldn't think about marrying me. I can't lie to you. I am not normal (she used the English word). You need to know this about me. And you should talk to your family—they will tell

you not to marry me." . . . And he said he wasn't worried about it. He said, "I'm an old man. If I end up dying of AIDS it's okay. I want to marry you."

In his analysis of what stigma is and how it operates, Erving Goffman (1963) laid out the complex set of unspoken rules the stigmatized are expected to learn and follow when interacting with "normals," such as acting as if one is normal (that is, not drawing attention to one's non-normalness) in order to protect "normals" from feeling uncomfortable, while simultaneously also subtly signaling that one is aware of one's non-normal state. As if taking a page straight from Goffman, Kelapi, like many people in Tari, drew a distinction between HIV-positive people and "normal" people, using the English word "normal" to refer to people presumed to be HIV-negative. And, as will be seen, the other women I interviewed also enacted some of the interactional rules identified by Goffman, particularly protecting "normals" in various ways and taking care not to be seen as trying to pass as "normal."

The English word "normal," which I had never heard used before in Tari, had become a semiotically dense category: it referred to an HIV-negative sero-status, but it was also about having a "normal" body (that is, looking HIV-negative, based on stereotypes about HIV-positive people being thin and weak), having a hazard-free body (as opposed to the HIV-positive, who were sometimes spoken of as contaminating or polluting), and being morally reliable (as opposed to the HIV-positive, who were often considered morally suspect). Given the social safety of being "normal," it was not surprising that the women I interviewed often expressed an acute longing to *kamap normal* (become normal)—that is, to be cured of HIV— or to be *olsem normal* (like normal). To "become normal" was not only to be free of the virus, but also free of the moral blemish and danger associated with HIV; to be "like normal" was simply to be treated like everyone else, without one's HIV status overwhelming one's other characteristics. However, with no cure in sight, "becoming normal" was unlikely, and being "like normal" presented many challenges.

As discussed in chapter 5, many of the women were uncertain about how they would fare on ARVs in the long term, or whether the medicines would continue to be available. Some were coming to terms with a weaker body, less able to contribute labor to their households. Some had been widowed by AIDS, and others ostracized by family, and in either case, they were usually worse off economically than before. All of these circumstances meant that they often felt that being "like normal" was out of reach and that they instead had to learn how best to live with their non-normal status (see also Mattes 2014). Some, like Kelapi (or Gloria, from chapter 5), thrived on ARVs and felt a renewed sense of strength, vigor, and purpose, but even these women had to confront questions about their ethical obligations to others given that they were HIV-positive. Kelapi, for example, was reluctant to expose her fiancé to the risk of becoming HIV-positive or to the disapproval of his family. Accommodating themselves to and managing others' fears and suspicions also made the ability to live "like normal" nearly impossible for most women.

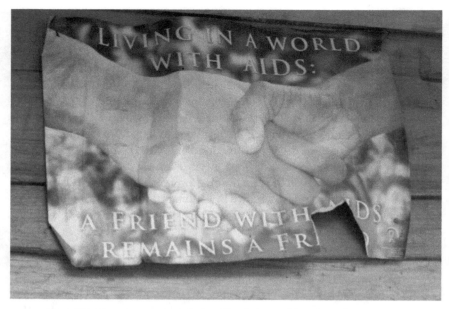

FIGURE 8. AIDS awareness poster on the outside of a house. Photo by author.

In chapter 5, I focused on how HIV-positive women care for themselves, often keeping an apprehensive eye on their own interior emotional states. In this chapter, I examine how they strive to act as moral persons, often by anticipating others' (often illusory) fears about AIDS and seeking to protect them. Because AIDS is stigmatized and associated with moral wrongdoing, the newly diagnosed face HIV, not only as a health problem, but also as a moral problem. To maintain others' forbearance and goodwill, they must demonstrate that they are "the good kind of HIV-positive person"—not the kind that might hide their status and infect others. And, given their dependence on others, and in some cases their isolation and reduced means, they must determine how to forge ethical lives in a society that values generosity, reciprocity, and exchange relations above all.

THE MORAL PROBLEM OF BEING HIV-POSITIVE

In the early 2000s, the stigma attached to AIDS was blatant, and the consequences were sometimes brutal. There were stories in Tari of infected people confined in pig houses, tied to trees and left out at night in the rain, or taken into the bush and abandoned, much as reported in the Eastern Highlands (Hammar 2010). How widespread such responses may have been is impossible to know, but the stories demonstrate the fear, revulsion, and moral opprobrium associated with AIDS at that time. Since 2007, the generally very good access to ARVs in the Tari area has dramatically lessened the fear and stigma associated with HIV and has changed how stigma is expressed (cf. Castro and Farmer 2005). Almost all of the women I interviewed reported feeling healthy most of the time and were usually able to carry out some or most of the labor expected of women. No longer wasting away, and now able to do agricultural and household work, they were accepted by their families. And, because they looked "normal" they were treated "like normal" by their immediate family members, if not always by extended family or the wider community.

Widespread AIDS education, as well as the expectation that treatment support-ers accompany patients to clinic appointments, have also played important roles in decreasing stigma. The women I interviewed were usually the most knowledgeable about HIV/AIDS in their households, but could not presume to act as the fam-ily educator. Consequently, they appreciated the "rule" that treatment support-ers had to accompany a patient to her clinic appointments because it forced the accompanying family members to be educated about HIV when otherwise they might have retained incorrect knowledge that caused fear and justified exclusion-ary practices. Acquiring accurate information about transmission made family members far more willing to share housing, food, blankets, utensils, and clothing with patients. Thus, while policy makers may imagine that patients should have treatment supporters in order to ensure that they adhere to their medications, the female patients I interviewed saw their "treatment supporters" as a kind of captive clinic audience receiving accurate and destigmatizing health information.

This is not to say that equipping people with biomedically correct knowledge about HIV perfectly rectified mistreatment: one-third of the women I interviewed had been ostracized and treated cruelly, sometimes violently, by family members. For almost all of them, this was because their sexual reputations had been tar-nished prior to their HIV diagnosis: they had "passengered around" before or during marriage, they had attended *dawe anda,* or they had run off to marry a hus-band their family disapproved of. In these cases, accurate information about AIDS did not dispel family feelings of disgust or disapproval, or their belief that an HIV-positive person was dirty and contaminating. For example, Shelly, discussed in chapter 5, had two older brothers who were convinced that she had infected herself and then her husband by "passengering around," and she avoided going to a par-ticular roadside market where she was likely to encounter one brother because he had once loudly announced, when she sat down next to him, "Look at this AIDS woman sitting next to me! She had better leave because I can smell the stench of her AIDS coming out of her vagina and getting on my skin." She didn't think her brother actually believed that HIV could be spread in this miasmatic way; rather, this was how he expressed his repugnance and his desire to humiliate her. His insult drew on long-standing Huli discourses about sexual pollution in which women's bodily fluids and smells are said to "block men's noses" or "get on their skin" and thereby damage their well-being and future fortunes (Glasse 1974, Frankel 1980, Clark 1993). While village court cases and demands for compen-sation for women's "menstrual pollution" are much rarer now than in the past (Wardlow 2006a), the idioms and ideas that informed them—about the connections between women's moral infractions, their bodily emanations, and others' illness—continue to have purchase, fueling misgivings about HIV-positive people, especially women.

Nevertheless, ARVs and AIDS education have significantly diminished AIDS dread by producing healthy, able bodies and by providing people with accurate information about transmission. But AIDS stigma derives not only from fears of death or physical contamination; it is also an act of judgment about a person's moral nature, intentions, and possible future acts, and ARVs have not diminished the suspicions that many people hold about the HIV-positive: that they brought infection upon themselves through moral transgression, that they must therefore deserve the punishment of HIV, and that their sexual misdeeds are indicative of broader moral flaws. For example, it is often said of women reputed to be passenger women that they also drink, smoke, gamble, refuse to do agricultural work, are more likely to lie and steal, were rebellious when young, had undisciplined upbringings, and come from bad families. Learning that someone is HIV-positive thus immediately raises doubts, suspicions, and sometimes a priori judgments, about her past behavior and moral makeup.

By the late 2000s, AIDS stigma was more subtly expressed. Public insults were far rarer than they had been, people said, but still occurred. For example, Jennifer, a young woman who had recently given birth to an HIV-negative baby, said that during her pregnancy women cruelly speculated aloud as to what she might give birth to (a frog? a snake? a rotting fetus?), and after the birth commented that it was unnatural and unfair that she had given birth to a healthy, "normal" child. She tried to control her reaction to these cruel comments because she did not want to give in to dangerous angry feelings. Her rejoinder (which other women I interviewed also articulated) was: "You can say what you want now, but AIDS can come just as easily to you. Tomorrow you could be next." Given the vicious and obscene insults that women typically exchange when angry, I was initially nonplussed by this seemingly tepid retort and by the pride my interlocutors clearly felt about it. I eventually came to understand that this was a quite calculated response: it did not reach the level of insult that could be characterized as "describing" a woman (that is, insulting her by talking about her body or her sexual reputation), which might invite retaliatory violence, but was instead intended to get under her skin and cause lingering worry by undermining her confidence in her husband's sexual fidelity. It was a way of evening the discursive playing field by emphasizing that all married women were vulnerable to a husband's philandering. Anyone might be next.

Public insults were less common than before, women said, for two reasons. First, local leaders had made a point of educating their communities about the HAMP (HIV/AIDS Management and Prevention) Act, which forbids publicly shaming an HIV-positive person: "The term 'stigmatise' is defined and includes 'to vilify or incite hatred, ridicule or contempt against a person or group on the grounds of an attribute,'" Genevieve Howse explains (2008: 4). Public verbal insults such as those directed at Jennifer, Shelly, or Rosina (see chapter 5) were, in fact, violations of the HAMP Act. Second, people feared that they might become vulnerable to demands for homicide compensation if they insulted an HIV-positive person who subsequently died. People living with HIV/AIDS had been known to commit suicide, and others had died even while taking ARVs, deaths that were often attributed to lethal worry. In either case an insulter could be accused of being a *tene* (cause) of the person's death. Consequently, stigma was more often demonstrated through such behaviors as passing an HIV-positive person on the road and refusing to look at or speak to her (*ngui higibi* in Huli; *pulim nus* in Tok Pisin), refusing to buy a woman's produce at market, or discontinuing small, daily exchange relations, such as sharing cigarettes, betel nut, or soft drinks. Noticeably, these might all be characterized as inactions, rather than actions, making them less easily targeted by laws like the HAMP Act.

More egregious instances of inaction included refusing to help an HIV-positive person rebuild a house, prepare land for planting, or assist in paying children's school fees. The women I interviewed who had young children worried constantly that if they died, no one would assist in paying their school fees or that greedy kin might try to appropriate land to which their children had a rightful claim. They also worried that people would simply be cruel. As Shelly said,

> I do this (adhere to her medication) for my children. If I die, it doesn't matter to me (*mi dai, nogat samting*). But my children—if I die people will say terrible things to them like, "This AIDS woman gave birth to you. You are not our child. Go cry on her grave." And they won't take care of them. So that's how I strengthen my control over my thoughts. I think of my two children. Who will take care of them if I fall down dead?

Even women who were seen as victims of their husbands' wayward behavior suffered some degree of stigma in the form of skepticism about their moral intentions. Perhaps counterintuitively, such skepticism was in part a consequence of ARVs. Indeed, many HIV-negative people (or presumably HIV-negative people, since most had not been tested) expressed ambivalence about the medications provided to those living with HIV. ARVs were lauded because they had saved loved ones from death, allowed them to live productive lives, and had largely rendered nonexistent the abject and frightening body of the person dying from AIDS-related illnesses. However, ARVs were also widely spoken of with suspicion, and even condemnation, as enabling HIV-positive people to "pass as normal (*giaman olsem normal*)." To *giaman* is to lie or pretend. For example, when someone gives false testimony at a village court case, other people often stand up and loudly yell, *Em giaman!* (He's lying!). And when older women laugh about flirting with a man, they may say, *Mi giaman olsem mi kamap sixteen gen* (I acted like I was sixteen again). To *giaman olsem normal*, however, is not just to playfully pretend to be something; it is to duplicitously try to pass as something one isn't, possibly for malevolent reasons.

For many people—men in particular, it seemed to me—the arrival of ARVs in Tari blurred what they believed to have been a clear and visible distinction between the HIV-positive and the HIV-negative. Despite much AIDS education to the contrary, there was still a common misperception that you could, in fact, tell if someone was HIV-positive by looking at them. Many of the women I interviewed, for example, had been sexually propositioned by men who refused to believe they were HIV-positive because they looked healthy. They sometimes had to show these men their clinic books and medications to convince them. Consequently, many people—again, men in particular—asserted that ARVs had a questionable effect, which was that they prevented the easy identification of HIV-positive people by making them look *olsem normal*. In rural Malawi, Amy Kaler, Nicole Angotti, and Astha Ramaiya noted similar "anxieties about the possibility that women on treatment, who appear healthy, may actually be dangerous to men seeking a wife, a steady girlfriend or a casual partner, because treatment restores the body to a healthy appearance, thus concealing evidence of infection," and ARVs were thus seen as "good for individuals" but a "danger to the community" (Kaler et al. 2016: 71, 74). In Tari, people sometimes said that ARVs made it possible for an HIV-positive person to *giaman olsem normal* and to *spreim sik AIDS* (spray AIDS) or *spredim sik AIDS* (spread AIDS). The English words "spray" and "spread"—perhaps introduced by health workers—had entered Huli vocabulary and were used interchangeably and conjoined, so that to "spray" or "spread" AIDS referred both to the spurting of dangerous sexual substances and the transmission of HIV.

Exacerbating this fear was that people living with HIV were sometimes spoken of as essentially, biologically different, and this was attributed to HIV being "a disease of the blood" (*sik bilong blat*), an idiom introduced by health workers, not anticipating how this might be taken up and interpreted. HIV changed the blood of those who were infected, some people said, so that the HIV-positive not only had dangerous bodies, but also harbored dangerous emotions and desires. Attributing intentionality and agency to the virus, some people said that because the virus wanted to spread itself to many bodies, it increased sexual desire in those it infected. Others said that having an incurable virus made people angry—angry enough to lash out and force others to join them by seducing or sexually assaulting them. After the arrival of good access to ARVs and widespread education, such ideas were losing purchase in the popular imagination. Nevertheless, it was a worrying paradox for some people that the same medicines that could "fence in" or "fight against" HIV might also make its spread more likely by camouflaging those who had it.

Giaman olsem normal *and Being Morally Suspect*

Because of doubts about the characters of people living with HIV and ambiguous perceptions of ARVs, the women I interviewed found themselves inhabiting a liminal moral status—they were not perceived as morally bad, but as morally suspect, not quite trustworthy. This status often necessitated that they behave in ways that would continually reassure others about their benign intentions. They often felt they were walking a fine line between trying to *stap olsem normal* (live like normal) while making it clear that they were not trying to *giaman olsem normal* (pass as normal). Despite their stated desires *not* to stand out as exceptional or different, they had to perpetually interpellate themselves as HIV-positive, to reflect self-consciously on the implications of this essentialized difference, and to show others that they acknowledged it and acted accordingly. And since Huli women are typically dependent on others for housing, food, and protection, they often had to live in such a way that others believed they were worthy of care. Many spoke of trying to achieve a less suspect status by performing an exaggerated version of female morality.

Hygienic Morality.   A common practice of the women I interviewed was what I call hygienic morality—that is, they created and policed boundaries between themselves and other household members in order to guarantee that they would not infect them. Many of them said that household members were happy to "finish my Coca Cola" or "share my blanket," but they also spoke of not permitting family members to do so. If they had their own rooms or mattresses, they would not allow children or their sisters to sleep with them, despite the normalcy of this sleeping arrangement and their own desires for this companionship. Similarly, they insisted on having their own set of utensils, cup, and plate, which they alone ate from and washed. Such boundary-drawing behavior is reminiscent of Huli women's bodily comportment during menstruation, when women protect those around them by not handling food, not stepping over household objects, and even minimizing speech, so that their exhalations won't affect others. Although none of the women I interviewed explicitly articulated parallels between menstrual pollution and HIV, it seemed that they drew on moral practices from the former domain to inform the management of their bodies with respect to the latter.

Since both they and their household members knew that HIV could not be transmitted through these modes of sharing, these acts of boundary-drawing were intended by the women, and taken by their families, as demonstrations of their commitment to protecting and caring for others. Indeed, an HIV-positive woman and her family often engaged in an ethical pas de deux in which the woman would demonstrate her love and care for them by establishing spatial boundaries around herself and objects she touched, and they would demonstrate their love and care for her by violating these boundaries—drinking from her cup, borrowing her clothes, and so on. They knew that these boundaries were biomedically unnecessary, and that she was demonstrating her intent to protect them, and she knew that their boundary-crossing was intended to show her that they were not afraid and trusted her. In a sense, information about how HIV could not be transmitted (by sharing cups, spoons, clothes) was mobilized by family members in a subtle dance of love and care.

HIV-positive women's care-taking and hygienic morality carried over into public settings, such as the roadside markets where women often sell produce or cooked food. For example, this was how Gloria (who, as we saw in chapter 5, asserted that she now lived better than she had when her husband was alive) described how she prepared herself when going to the market:

> I wash myself thoroughly before I sell things in the market. I tie my hair up and cover it. Only then do I carry my produce to market, and then people aren't afraid of me. I think to myself that I must stay healthy and I must look healthy. I must look like all of them. So I wash well, and I arrange my hair. I clip my nails. And I wear gloves. I make sure my clothes look nice and clean and don't have tears or stains. And I make sure that if I'm selling cooked food that it is covered well with a cloth. And I always bring a fork or some tongs, and I use them to serve people. I never touch the food with my hands when I'm at the market. I make sure the food is in a good clean bowl. [It sounds like you have thought of everything and that you arrive at the market really prepared.] Yes, I think of everything. I think that if I go to market I cannot look as if I am sick. I must look completely normal. That way people will think, "Yes, we know she's sick. But she looks healthy and clean, so we can buy from her."

There is a tension here between Gloria's desire to be perceived as "normal" and the elaborate and atypical practices she undertakes in order to achieve this. In other words, in order to be accepted as normal, Gloria, and many of the other women I interviewed, adopted exceptional—that is, "abnormal"—practices. For example, Gloria demonstrates exaggerated care about hygiene. Although women generally make sure that their produce is well washed for market display, they do not cover their hair, clip their nails, wear gloves, or use tongs to handle food. Gloria does these things, not only to assure people that her food is safe, but also to advertise to them that she is the kind of HIV-positive woman who has reflected on her sero-status and is taking care to minimize any hazard they think she might pose. In other words, she is both protecting others and making her intent to protect them visible. And, though she used the word "normal" to describe the impression she was trying to achieve, in fact Gloria is not striving to "pass" as "normal"; rather, by setting herself apart from other women at the market with her rigorously hygienic behavior, she is semiotically mobilizing information about how HIV is *not* transmitted to establish her ethical intentions.

Absolute Candor.   One might wonder how the people at the market knew that Gloria was HIV-positive. This is likely because of another ethical practice that many of the women I interviewed stressed: absolute candor about their HIV-positive status. AIDS policy makers have encouraged open disclosure about HIV, the logic being that secrecy only reinforces exceptionalism, stigma, and shame, while candor contributes to normalization and stigma reduction. Nevertheless, the existing public health and anthropological research suggests that people living with HIV exercise cautious deliberation about whom to tell and whom not to tell, and typically disclose their HIV status to few people in order to avoid stigma, or simply to preserve their existing identities and social belonging (Bond 2010, Hardon and Posel 2012, Mattes 2012). In contrast, almost all the women I interviewed said that they had disclosed their sero-status to neighbors and clan members, as well as to close and extended family members, and had even announced it at local markets and other large community venues, such as before weekly village court cases or before church services began. I was repeatedly told, "Everyone knows, everyone in my community knows."

The most common reason women gave for this practice of wide disclosure was that they recognized that for some community members (though certainly not all), not informing others of one's HIV-positive status was equivalent to hiding it. Remaining silent about one's sero-status left open the possibility that one was trying to *giaman olsem normal,* which cast one's moral intentions into doubt. Ethical behavior thus entailed, not only not infecting others, but also assertively and widely disclosing one's status in order to prevent others' suspicions about one's possible malevolent intentions. As a number of women stated plainly, "Only people who want to spread/spray it around don't reveal their status to everyone." In openly confessing or avowing their HIV-positive status, women were likely informed by a Christian tradition. Most of them belonged to a Christian denomination and had grown up going to church, and as HIV patients, they had received counselling about the importance of disclosing their HIV status to others (Nguyen 2013), though I never witnessed any health workers urging patients to make public declarations. Again, the desire to live one's life "like normal" came into conflict with the possibility of being perceived as trying to "pass" as normal, and in the end many women chose active and widespread disclosure as both the most ethical and self-protective path.

Women's commitment to candor extended to men who propositioned them, though they typically had mixed motives, both wanting to protect the men from HIV and wanting to protect themselves from unwanted advances. Men might be looking for a one-off sexual encounter, a girlfriend, or a wife, but whatever their intentions, almost all the women I interviewed said that they were regularly sexually propositioned. All but a couple of the women asserted that they uniformly rejected these proposals and, moreover, informed the propositioners of their HIV-positive status. For example, Betty—a middle-aged woman who had fled to a *dawe anda* after two very violent marriages, and who continued to attend *dawe anda* post-diagnosis, despite the damage this did to her reputation—had this to say about her HIV candor:

> [So did you tell your family when you found out your diagnosis?] Yes, I told them. I told everyone. I told it everywhere. [Everywhere?] Yes, everywhere—if someone asks me, I tell him/her yes. [Do you mean like if men ask you?] Yes, yes! Men often ask

me to have sex with them, and I say, "No, I have HIV." [And how do they respond?] Many of them accuse me of lying and making excuses. [So what do you do?] I always carry around my medicine and my clinic book, and I show them. I say, "Look, here in my clinic book it says I have AIDS. Look, here is my AIDS medicine." Lots of men have propositioned me, and they say, "But you don't look like an AIDS woman. You look healthy—let's go have sex at a guesthouse." And I say, "No, sorry, good man. I am an AIDS woman. I am a dead woman. Look at my clinic book. Look at my medicine."

Women typically used the phrases "I am an AIDS woman" (*mi AIDS meri*) or "My blood is ruined" (*blad bilong mi bagarap finis*), or even "I am already dead" (*mi dai finis*), to deter their propositioners. While this language arguably reinforced AIDS stigma—and perhaps reflects a degree of internalized abjection—it was also effective in driving away unwanted advances. When such self-descriptors failed, women resorted to the kinds of demonstrations described by Betty or even, in a couple of cases, to announcing loudly for anyone nearby to hear, "I have AIDS, and this man is propositioning me!"

MORAL LUCK, BURDENED VIRTUES, AND BEING AN HIV-POSITIVE WOMAN

The moral logic employed in many of the women's narratives tended towards what might be called a deontological ethical orientation; in other words, women indicated that their morality was guided by and would be judged according to whether they abided by particular rules, duties, and obligations. In the field of moral philosophy, ethical theories are often divided into three rough schools of thought: deontological ethics, which emphasizes norms and rules; virtue ethics, which focuses on the cultivation of virtues, character, and moral reasoning; and consequentialist ethics, which privileges the harmful or beneficial consequences of an act in determining its moral value. Much recent anthropological work has adopted a virtue ethics approach (Laidlaw 2002; Zigon 2009; Lambek 2010a, 2010b; Mattingly 2014; Das 2015). In contrast, the women I interviewed emphasized a range of duties and obligations: to protect others from the (often illusory) threat of their bodies, to protect family from compensation demands that might ensue from their HIV-positive status, and to avoid any appearance of duplicity about their sero-status. Categorizing my interlocutors' practices into one school of moral thought or another is, admittedly, a tricky undertaking since, for example, cultivating obedience to particular rules would likely be considered a virtue for Huli women. And, as Didier Fassin notes, "in 'real world' situations that anthropologists examine, when they attempt to comprehend the moral arguments expressed by individuals to justify their actions or the ethical practices performed by them in the course of their everyday life, it is seldom possible to sort out the deontological, virtuous, and consequentialist threads" (Fassin 2015: 8). Nevertheless, it is worth considering why the women I interviewed put such emphasis on rules and obligations.

First, it should be noted that Huli moral philosophy might be said to have a deontological cast—that is, people often emphasize the importance of moral injunctions, taboos, and duties, and this is especially true for women. Women have long been figured as needing to be "fenced in" by specific rules and by the disciplinary practices of others (especially brothers and husbands) in order to behave morally. Without forceful—which is to say, physically punitive—socialization about gendered rules of conduct, women are thought likely to become "wayward" (Wardlow 2006a). That said, I believe that many Huli would assert that no one, male or female, can cultivate a virtuous character without first prioritizing moral rules. Everyone needs to be "fenced in," and rules, taboos, duties, and obligations are the fences.[3] Indeed, one of the problems with the modern era, people say, is that "we are no longer fenced in."

As important as the deontological tendencies in Huli moral thought is the positionality of the women I interviewed. That they were gendered female and viewed as not "normal" strongly shaped their moral reasoning and acts. The work of feminist moral philosophers helps to elucidate how being female, socioeconomically dependent, and morally suspect pushed them to think about their actions in terms of moral duties. While the field of moral philosophy has traditionally posited an ahistorical, context-free, autonomous ethical subject who can freely choose his or her course of action, feminist philosophers have made a point of considering the effect that a subject's socially structured position might have on his or her ethical capacity, reasoning, and conduct. For example, Claudia Card, in her book *The Unnatural Lottery* (1996), took the philosophical concept of "moral luck" (Williams 1981, Nagel 1993)—a situation where circumstances beyond one's control affect one's moral actions—and argued for the necessity of considering "circumstances that are *systematically* arranged and that tend to affect people as members of social groups" (Tessman 2000: 377, emphasis in original). In other words, she urged moral philosophers to conceptualize "luck" not as haphazard circumstances, but rather as robust, structuring inequalities, such as class, race, and gender. She referred to these as "the unnatural lottery" because, as she explained, the "lottery" of one's life chances could not be considered random or "natural" when they were partially determined by skin color, sexed body, and so on.

The moral problems Card examines using the concept of moral luck consequently diverge significantly, for example, from the question of whether two equally attentive and skilled drivers should be morally assessed in the same way when one of them suffers the unfortunate circumstance of having a dog run across the road, causing her to swerve and fatally hit people (this is a classic example often used to explain the concept of moral luck). Rather, Card asks how gender inequality, gendered violence, and what is now sometimes called "rape culture" affect women's ability to live fully flourishing ethical lives. She also develops the concept of "moral damage"—that is, the ways in which abusive contexts can have limiting or distorting effects on a subject's moral reasoning and judgment.

Lisa Tessman, building on Card's work, focuses on how experiencing systemic marginalization or oppression, such as racism, shapes the moral self: "The first and most obvious way is that it creates circumstances external to the oppressed agent . . . that limit options so that every way one turns one runs into barriers that make it difficult or impossible to gain or be granted freedom, material resources, political power, and respect or social recognition of personhood—all of which are needed to live well" (Tessman 2000: 375). When she says that these things are needed "to live well," she is referring to Aristotle's concept of *eudaimonia,* a key concept in virtue ethics, which has been variably translated as human flourishing, self-cultivation, self-actualization, or the pursuit of excellence. In order to differentiate her work from that of classical, Aristotelian or neo-Aristotelian virtue ethics, and to signal her attention to structures of inequality, Tessman characterizes her own work as *critical* virtue ethics (Tessman 2001). A critical virtue ethics, she says, examines the specific ways that exclusion, violence, discrimination, and precarity not only limit a subject's *socioeconomic* opportunities, or damage her *psychological* well-being, but also cause harm to her as a *moral* actor, constraining her chances of achieving *eudaimonia.* Her aim, Tessman says, is "to name moral limitations and burdens as belonging on a list of harms that oppression causes, and to express both anger and grief over these harms" (Tessman 2005: 5).

By moral harm or damage Tessman does not mean that an actor will engage in unethical acts that she wouldn't have otherwise; rather, there is a certain sort of a self that one ought to be, but the unconducive conditions of oppression bar one from cultivating this self. In an Aristotelian schema, such moral damage in turn disqualifies one from flourishing, for virtue is necessary for flourishing (Tessman 2005:4).

In other words, because a subject has not come into herself in a context of security or inclusion, she cannot fully act as the moral self that she might have become if she had lived with greater social justice and equality. She has not had the opportunity to cultivate the virtues, moral reasoning, and judgment that she might have. Crucially, it is also possible, even likely, that she has developed other virtues that have helped her endure her situation of oppression or discrimination. Tessman calls these "burdened virtues," which she defines as "a set of virtues that, while practically necessitated for surviving oppression or morally necessitated for opposing it, carry with them a cost to their bearer" (Tessman 2005: 4).

One of Tessman's examples of a burdened virtue is anger about oppression, and she discusses the many ways in which anger can be a virtue, drawing on work by Audre Lorde, Elizabeth Spelman, and others (Tessman 2005: 117–23; see also chapter 5). "Focused with precision [anger] can become a powerful source of energy serving progress and change," Lorde observes (1984: 127), and Spelman argues that anger at an oppressor is an assertion of equality, because it constitutes a judgment of the oppressor's actions, and thus implicitly conveys that one has assumed the right to judge. "I am acting as if I have as much right to judge him as he assumes he has to judge me" (Spelman 1989: 266). That said, Tessman notes that anger is often a "burden": its expression can trigger retaliation from the oppressor; it can become painfully consuming as one comes to understand the intractable nature of oppression; or it can be misdirected "at others subject to the same mistreatments as oneself" (Tessman 2005: 122; cf. Lorde 1984). In short, burdened virtues come at a steep cost to the self and do not necessarily, or even often, contribute to *eudaimonia,* the subject's human flourishing. Rather, they emerge, become necessary, and are cultivated precisely because of the need to survive and sometimes to resist structures of stigma and oppression.

Hygienic morality, absolute candor, and other steps HIV-positive Huli women take to make others feel safe might also be considered burdened virtues. They often described their unusual practices as "rules I made for myself"; as discussed above, their discursive framing suggested a deontological slant in their approach to ethical behavior—an emphasis on rules, obligations, and imperatives. However, drawing on Tessman's work, I think one can see their practices as virtues that come at a cost to them, and that they cultivate in order to endure their reduced, dependent, and stigmatized circumstances. Taking precautions against being perceived as *giaman olsem normal,* for example, was a virtue that enabled women to be accepted by family and community; it demonstrated to others that one was a "good" HIV-positive person who was committed to protecting others. But this virtue was heavily "burdened": a woman had to be willing to repeatedly rehearse her difference from others through practices such as radical HIV disclosure. In essence, she had to sacrifice being "like normal," which is what most of the women longed for, to persuade others she wasn't trying to pass as normal. Similarly, biting one's tongue and walking away from people who were publicly insulting one prevented an altercation that might result in one's kin having to pay compensation, but it was humiliating and often came at a great cost to a woman's sense of dignity.

When considering why HIV-positive women have developed these burdened virtues, two factors emerge: (1) the atomism and lack of social support they experience, and (2) the pervasive violence in Tari. As observed in chapter 5, it is notable that there are no AIDS support groups in Tari, and there have been next to no efforts to bring people living with HIV together, to enable their greater self-reliance, or to assist them in reflecting critically on their shared experiences. One question I asked everyone I interviewed was whether they knew other HIV-positive people or had HIV-positive friends, and many said that although they had met others at the clinic, they only ever saw them when they came to pick up their medication every three months. A few women expressed a desire to live with women they had met at the clinic, but none could imagine a way for this to be possible, given that they didn't own their own houses or land. In other words, women's material dependencies not only make them more vulnerable to HIV, but also make it more difficult for them to form networks of care once they are HIV-positive.

Some of the anthropological literature about HIV support groups has stressed how they operate as nodes in the global AIDS governmental assemblage, enforcing "the rules" of ART adherence, making access to ARVs contingent on group membership, strongly shaping the confessional narratives members tell about their intimate lives, policing each other's conduct, and, in tandem with HIV counselling, producing obedient responsibilized patient-subjects (Colvin et al. 2010, Mattes 2011, Mfecane 2011, Prince 2012). This literature is often skeptical of support groups, despite their intended function of enabling mutual assistance and community. That said, support groups have also been analyzed as sites for combatting public and internalized stigma (Beckman and Bujra 2010, Liamputtong et al. 2009, Paudel and Baral 2015), creating greater self-sufficiency (White and Morton 2005), and forging critical consciousness-raising and solidarity (Lyttleton 2004, Robins 2006). The absence of such groups in Tari meant not only that my interlocutors typically had no friends who shared their situation, but also that they felt no sense of solidarity around the issues of HIV stigma or precarity. Rather, they usually felt very alone in their experiences of living with HIV. And, alone in their situations, and often dependent on kin, they felt compelled to prove that they were doing all they could to behave as moral HIV-positive persons who were worthy of care.

Violence also shaped women's moral reasoning and acts. Most of the women knew about cases of violence towards people living with AIDS during the pre-ARVs era, and were aware that some kin and neighbors continued to harbor fear and suspicion of HIV-positive people. Women's own personal experiences of violence must also be taken into account when analyzing how they understood themselves as ethical subjects. Whether raped by their husband, like Kelapi, or raped during an armed holdup of a PMV, like Sarah (see chapter 2), many of the women had been victims of sexual violence. Most had also experienced violence in their marriages, and many had experienced injury at the hands of brothers and other family members. Physical violence—whether inflicted by kin, criminals, or clan enemies—was never far away for anyone in Tari, but women were particularly vulnerable, and, because of the fear and suspicion associated with HIV, a positive diagnosis only exacerbated this vulnerability. Women living with family worried about the consequences of making household members angry (being evicted), and women living alone worried about home invasion. And, all of them were well aware that, as discussed in chapter 2, interpersonal violence could quickly escalate into "trouble"—that is, political violence—as threatened to happen in Rosina's case (see chapter 5), when insults traded over a basketball game became a physical fight between people from different families and clans.

Dependence on family and a context of pervasive interpersonal, political, and gendered violence intersected to shape women's moral behavior. For many, their uncertain and tenuous positions in their households forced them to think about how best to maintain others' indulgence and care. For example, some made a point of providing as much domestic and agricultural labor as their health allowed.

Most important, their dependence and fear of violence created two overarching moral imperatives for them: (1) do not *giaman olsem normal,* and (2) do not bring "trouble" to one's family. By following these imperatives, they hoped to avoid the possibility of punitive violence (from family) or retaliatory violence (from non-family) should they be accused of infecting others. Whether we want to call women's allegiance to self-imposed rules a tendency to deontology or a burdened virtue, this allegiance emerged from their specific positionality of being female and HIV-positive in a context where physical violence was pervasive and there were few supports for people living with HIV/AIDS apart from family.

THE HIGHEST VIRTUE: GIVING

A number of ethnographers have analyzed the challenges of trying to live a "normal" life when living with HIV. Dominik Mattes, for example, casts a skeptical eye on global health discourses that assert that ARVs enable patients to resume a normal life, noting that in Tanzania, "'normalcy' entailed more than mere bodily reconstitution. It implied . . . .rehabilitated social and economic relations, resumed sexual activity, and a reconstituted sense of self" (Mattes 2014: 271), all of which were almost impossible to achieve in a context of precarity and continuing HIV stigma. Mattes observes that the hallmark of "normal" life, marrying and having children, was the biggest challenge because it "confronted patients with the basically unresolvable moral dilemma that this was only possible at the cost of accepting the risk of infecting one's partner" (283). While marriage and childbearing are also markers of normalcy among the Huli, equally important is being enmeshed in relations of giving and reciprocity. In the language of virtue ethics, generosity, the skillful expansion of one's social networks, and acumen in contributing materially to others' endeavors are all virtues to be cultivated through practice, self-sacrifice, reflection, and the discerning observation of how others conduct their own exchange relationships. Indeed, these could be said to be the most important virtues for *eudaimonia*—human flourishing.

Relations of reciprocity and exchange have been emphasized in the ethnographic literature about Papua New Guinea so often that its inhabitants have come to serve as exemplars of these cultural traits, "an anthology of images in and through which anthropologists have frozen the contribution of specific cultures to our understanding of the human condition," constituting a "language of incarceration" (Appadurai 1988: 36–37). Most anthropology students are familiar, for example, with the competitive, ceremonial exchange of pigs and other wealth items in the Highlands of Papua New Guinea (Strathern 1971) or the kula ring of the Trobriand islands, in which men canoe from one island to another to exchange prized items (Malinowski 1922). Probably almost as familiar are practices of bridewealth or homicide compensation—the giving of pigs, money, shells, and other valuables to a group that has lost one of its members, whether through marriage or death.

What has been less emphasized in the ethnographic literature (but see Lederman 1986) are the little gifts—sweet potatoes, betel nut, cigarettes, fresh greens, an item of secondhand clothing, a small piece of roast pork, boiled chicken feet, flavor sachets from an instant noodle soup packet, a couple of kina, "flex cards" (mobile phone credit vouchers)—that make up everyone's days, especially women's. Before leaving home, most women I know try to put a few such items in their string bags, knowing that they are likely to run into friends or kin to whom they should give something, no matter how small. And this ethos of daily giving is actively socialized: the first words taught to children are *ngi* (give me) and *ma* (here, take it), which are practiced over and over with various small objects until a toddler readily gives up what she has when asked, and takes what is given to her. Children who display selfishness or lack of gratitude are told sternly that if they aren't generous or fail to show appreciation for others' generosity, they will "have only their own shit to eat," a graphic reminder that hermetic individualism is pragmatically unwise and morally repugnant (Wardlow 2006). And, through witnessing their family members contribute to others' bridewealth and homicide payments, school fees, and plane tickets, children learn that it is through this regular give-and-take that one not only forges necessary networks of assistance but also cultivates a life that is affectively rich and morally meaningful. Underlying the large, competitive, ritual exchanges analyzed in much of the ethnographic literature, in other words, is a powerful, simple message learned when young—that one must give.

These daily small acts of giving can be seen as a mode of "ordinary ethics." Michael Lambek uses the term "ordinary ethics" (2010a and b) to signal that ethical sensibilities are intrinsic to everyday speech and action. Rather than understanding ethical decisions or acts as particular moments that punctuate the flow of normal life, Lambek sees ethical considerations as saturating this flow. Since social interaction entails the continuous, often subconscious, evaluation of others, as well as continual self-evaluation and self-adjustment to the (perceived) judgment of our actions by others, most of our social interactions, he suggests, entail ethical considerations. Moreover, "ordinary," for Lambek, "implies an ethics that is relatively tacit, grounded in agreement rather than rule, in practice rather than knowledge or belief, and happening without calling undue attention to itself" (Lambek 2010a: 2). All this well describes Huli women's daily practices of gift-giving.

For Veena Das, ordinary ethics are "small acts of everyday repair" or "textures of attentiveness in sustaining everyday life" (2015: 79); they are inconspicuous gestures that spare another's dignity or create a connection across difference. Das adds that in her notion of the everydayness of ordinary ethics, "the everyday is not simply the world of routines or habits but is shadowed by doubts that can become world annihilating" (2015: 86). Much as Das says, the pervasive nature of violence in Tari—and most people's daily unease that something brutal and frightening (a murder in the marketplace, a home invasion at night) could happen at any time— means that their lives are indeed "shadowed by doubts that can become world annihilating." The little gifts that serve as "small acts of everyday repair" may, of course, involve strategy and calculus, but they more often entail remembering who has been kind in the past or suffered recently from illness, upset, or loss.

The women I interviewed were often preoccupied with the ordinary ethics of how to manage their relations of reciprocity. Whether to share or keep what one had; to expand one's networks or contract them; to invite people inside their homes or not; to cadge food and cigarettes from others, knowing one couldn't reciprocate, or to go hungry and smoke-free—all these were dilemmas they mulled over. Their strategies for self-care often entered into these deliberations. Peony, for example, said that when her daughter had married, she had given away all of her *imane aka*, a specific item of bridewealth, usually a large sum of money, given to the bride's mother, which she is not expected share. When I pointed out that her behavior was unusual, she said,

> Yes, you are right. But my reasoning was that I am a sick woman, so I shouldn't keep this money for myself. I should share it with my kin. Then later, if I need help because I'm sick, they will help me. It could be that later I won't have the strength and I will need help. So it's good if I am generous with my kin now.

In contrast, Zoli, whose daughter was also HIV-positive (see chapter 5), said that when her kin asked her to contribute to bridewealth or compensation payments she would reply,

> "Oh, sorry! I can't. I've got this sickness. I'm a sick woman!" I don't help other people with this kind of thing. I just take care of myself and my daughter. How can I help them?! I just say to them, "Will I continue to live or will I die? I don't know. So don't ask me to help with troubles or with marriages." That's what I tell people.

Peony's generosity was only partially successful, though other factors played a complicating role. When I interviewed her in 2012, she said that when she and her husband were diagnosed, they had agreed that they would renew their faith in God together, attend church regularly, and strive to be good Christians. When I interviewed her again in 2013, she was living alone and said she felt hungry much of the time: "Hunger kills me. In the evening I walk around to see who has smoke coming from their house, and then I go to their door and say, 'I've come because I'm hungry.' And they give me some sweet potato and greens." Since our previous interview, she had burned down her husband's house after he abandoned her to marry another woman from the AIDS clinic. Consequently, she'd had to flee his clan land, had no access to the sweet potato fields she had planted, and couldn't easily benefit from exchange relations she had established and worked hard to maintain there.

The strategies adopted by Peony and Zoli suggest that women's decisions about whether to give generously to others are primarily pragmatic and aimed at preserving their own lives, but women also spoke of feeling ashamed about husbanding their meager resources rather than sharing them. Lucy, for example, told me she did not invite people into her house because she knew exactly how long her supply of tea and sugar would last if she rationed it for herself, and she had decided that being able to have this small pleasure outweighed the shame she felt about being ungenerous. Most important, many women were ashamed about being so often in the position of having to ask for care, rather than being able to give it, and about feeling unable to act as generously as they had been before becoming sick. For some this was because they tired more easily and so couldn't work as hard at agricultural labor. Others, evicted by their kin, no longer had the gardens that make possible women's generosity to each other: they didn't have produce to sell, and thus weren't able to buy the betel nut, packets of cheese twists, and other small items that sustain women's intimate ties with others. If daily generosities and the development of vibrant relations of exchange are key elements of *eudaimonia* in this context, then the inability to participate in these relations can be seen as a form of "moral damage" (Tessman 2005) caused by the material and social losses of being HIV-positive.

CONCLUSION

AIDS stigma is expressed in multiple ways in Tari—sometimes through insults, but more often through acts of neglect and refusal. It is also reinforced through the new language of "normal" in which women walk a fine line between *stap olsem normal* (living like normal) and being careful not to *giaman olsem normal* (try to pass as normal). Access to ARVs, widespread AIDS education, and the effective communication of laws like the HAMP Act have reduced fear of HIV-positive people and curtailed the violent forms of stigma that occurred in the past. Nevertheless, a tenacious dimension of AIDS stigma is a kind of moral uncertainty about the HIV-positive: can they be relied on to keep their HIV to themselves, as it were, and not infect others? This moral doubt is to some extent exacerbated by ARVs, in that they are understood as masking what would otherwise be obvious illness; they save and strengthen the body, and thereby hide the virus it harbors. This moral doubt is greatly intensified for women whose reputations were damaged pre-diagnosis by transgressive sexual practices, such as "passengering around." Moral doubt is a perception—or simply a feeling of apprehension or unease—on the part of those who presume themselves to be HIV-negative. Nevertheless, the stigma is projected onto the HIV-positive as a group and becomes their responsibility to manage, in the manner suggested by Erving Goffman (1963).

Acting to assuage others' concerns about their intentions becomes part of the moral habitus for some HIV-positive women. They disclose their status widely in order to assure people that they aren't hiding it, and then make a point of demonstrating to people that they aren't "that kind" of HIV-positive person—the kind that might spray/spread it—by presenting themselves as both the same as other women (e.g., they sell produce at the market), but also different (e.g., they make a point of creating a hygienic buffer between themselves and their customers). This strategy works well for women like Gloria, who said she lives better now than pre-diagnosis, or Kelapi, who found work as a teacher and forged a new, loving marriage. For others, however, like Shelly, who often slept under a tarp in people's fields, these steps are not enough to overcome the sexually spoiled identities they had pre-diagnosis. AIDS stigma "feeds upon, strengthens and reproduces existing inequalities" (Parker and Aggleton 2003: 13), in this case the inequality between women categorized as good and those considered wayward (Wardlow 2006a). Gloria, for example, was perceived as a victim of her husband's transgressions and was warmly embraced by her family. In Shelly's case, a positive diagnosis only served to confirm her brothers' conviction that she was immoral. HIV was seen as just deserts for what they assumed was her previous sexually transgressive behavior.

AIDS stigma can be understood as a form of "moral damage" in that it can grievously diminish and constrain women's ability to cultivate the virtues—such as those developed through rich relations of generosity and exchange—that constitute an important element of human flourishing in this context. The practices women develop to manage other people's concerns about them can be understood as "burdened virtues"—capacities and skills that are perceived as good by others, and that enable them to manage their social relations successfully, but that come at a cost. These costs may include the disclosure of one's HIV status, when one might rather tell only family members, and the regular demonstration to others that one is not the kind of HIV-positive person who should be feared.

EPILOGUE

Theresa lived near the AIDS Care Centre, and so I often ran into her in 2013, my final year of fieldwork for this project. During one of our chats she looked at me and said hesitantly, "I am feeling normal now. Normal. So I want to get a blood test." It took me a second to understand what she was implying. We were both silent. I think neither of us wanted to put her delicate hopes into words for fear they might be crushed. "To find out what?" I finally asked. She replied:

> Well, because I feel normal now. Before I had a small problem (that is, she had experienced some HIV-related symptoms), but now I'm feeling normal. So I just want to check my blood and find out. ["And the medicine?" I asked, because I was worried that if she was feeling "normal" she might have stopped taking her ARVs, a response that was not characteristic of the women I interviewed, but somewhat characteristic of the men.] Yes, I'm taking the medicine, but I feel normal now. And the members of my church all say I look normal and that I must be praying really well, and that God is hearing me because I look normal now. So I'll get a blood test, and then I can go to Australia and meet one of my phone friends. I'm sick of PNG. I want to move to Australia. So I need a blood test (she meant an HIV antibody test).

Theresa's family received regular payments from PJV for a large number of the pylons carrying electricity from Hides to Porgera, and through the payment meetings, and through living in Porgera for a few years, she had come to know some of the Australian PJV staff. She was very attractive, laughed easily, and spoke English well, despite not having completed many years of school, so I was only a little surprised to learn that she been able to parlay her PJV connections into a couple of male phone friends in Australia. One of them sent her money from time to time and had said he would pay her way to Australia. But she knew that even if he sponsored her by applying for a prospective marriage visa, she would almost certainly be denied if she was HIV-positive.

After she had left her Porgeran policeman husband and moved back to Tari, she had fallen into a lifestyle of partying with Huli politicians and businessmen, sometimes accepting invitations to stay with them at hotels in Mendi and Mt. Hagen. But upon testing HIV-positive, she had *senisim pasin bilong mi* (changed my ways): she took her medicine as directed, had given up smoking and drinking, wistfully said no to requests from her former businessman friends, brought the clinic nurses small gifts of food, had started going to church every week, had announced her HIV-positive status to the congregation, and even hosted small prayer groups in her home. And now she felt "normal." Wasn't it possible, she wondered, that she had, in fact, "become normal"? Only a blood test, she knew, could answer this. But she kept putting it off and putting it off, afraid of how she would feel if she still tested HIV-positive. It was better to keep her dreams of moving to Australia alive, even if it meant perpetual deferral.

Theresa's hope that she might have sero-converted to HIV-negative—a hope so precious and fragile that she didn't want to crush it by saying it plainly—was expressed by only a few of the women that I interviewed. Most accepted with resignation health workers' assertions that this was impossible until a biomedical cure was discovered. However, Theresa's feelings of vigor and well-being, her aspirations for the future, and her determination to sustain her hopeful state of mind—even if it meant denying certain inevitabilities—reflected the mood of many people in Hela in the early 2010s.

The construction of the LNG, the status of Hela as a new province, and the work of transforming Tari into a provincial capital meant that there were hundreds of jobs available. Tari's main market, though basically a huge stretch of mud strewn with trash and sucked-dry, spat-out sugarcane, bustled with hundreds of sellers and customers every day. PMVs went safely back and forth to Mendi and Mt. Hagen, and brought back astonishing new items for purchase: one year, wigs in various colors and styles seemed to be the fashion of the day for women. Tari had relied for decades on a temperamental hydroelectric plant built years before by missionaries, and it had finally given up the ghost in the late 2000s, leaving the town without power. But because Tari was now a provincial capital, PNG Power, the national electric company, was finally erecting power lines and connecting businesses and government buildings to the national grid. And, because of the well-paid jobs provided by the LNG, many households were able to buy small generators, which they used to turn a profit charging people's mobile phones. Other people had money to spend because businesses were buying up land on the fringes of Tari town with the aim of building bank branches, small fast-food shops, and even a car dealership. Word that Tari was the place to be for those with an entrepreneurial spirit had spread: I had long talks in my guesthouse with a hairdresser who had come all the way from Goroka by herself, hoping to find a site where she might establish her own business keeping provincial officials and their families looking stylish (she was not able to make a go of it). She could scarcely believe that Tari—with its few squat buildings and dirt roads—was even considered a town, let alone a provincial capital. Certainly, it resembled no provincial capital she had ever been to before.

But despite the elation of the moment, it was also a time of foreboding. Whenever I visited Hides or Nogoli (LNG project areas), people there expressed distrust, resentment, and censure. The expatriate LNG workers "hid inside" their fenced compounds, people said, and only came and went by vehicle. They never actually walked around and talked to local people, which the latter found both mystifying and insulting. The relocation packages were grossly insufficient, given that people were giving up their land and homes. Jobs with ExxonMobil or Oil Search were available only to those willing to bribe or do sexual favors for the men in charge of hiring—indeed, one friend of mine was informed by a gatekeeper to employment that not only would she be required to have sex with him, he also expected her to provide her cell phone number and some photos that he could share with friends. Long-haul trucks, too large for the narrow dirt roads, drove too fast, nearly killing people and raising clouds of dust that made them sick. Lots of money was being paid in underhanded ways to defuse dissent, but very little was being invested in community or women's development: "The men who set up roadblocks and threaten to sabotage the project get paid thousands of kina to disperse, and we get cooking demonstrations," one woman said scornfully. And, most worryingly, people were extremely unhappy about the landowner identification process, which they described as rushed, incomplete, and problematic (see also Main and Fletcher 2018). The identification of some clans as LNG project area landowners, and some not, was causing a great deal of frustration, which people predicted would only get worse once the gas was finally flowing and royalties were paid (or not paid, or paid to the wrong people). They were correct.

The LNG made its first shipment of gas in 2014, which meant that the first royalty payments should have been made to appropriate incorporated landowning groups (ILGs) shortly thereafter. However, the process of identifying landowner beneficiaries had "been stalled since 2010" because landowner identification had "become tied up in PNG's court system as a result of several legal claims" (Main and Fletcher 2018: 12). Thus, as of 2018, while some royalty payments had been made to landowning groups around the gas-conditioning plant in Port Moresby, none had been made in Hela, where the vast majority of landowners lived. Moreover, ExxonMobil insisted that it was the Papua New Guinea government's responsibility to resolve the various competing claims and to complete the landowner identification process (Rix 2018), while critics asserted that it was the responsibility of the state and the project operator (that is, ExxonMobil) together to carry

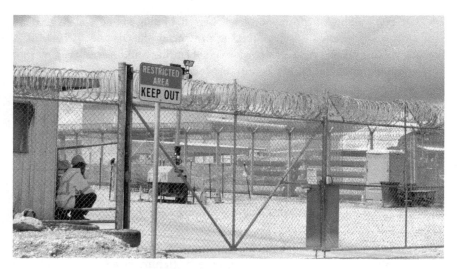

FIGURE 9. PNG LNG project site. Photo by Kenneth I. MacDonald.

out this process and assist landowners in organizing into ILGs so that they could "fairly and meaningfully enter into negotiations with the developers" (Main and Fletcher 2018: 12). Moreover, they said, this process should have been completed before breaking ground in 2009. As one might imagine, Hela landowner claimants have been extremely frustrated by these delays, particularly since the plentiful economic opportunities and benefits largely evaporated with the completion of the construction phase of the LNG.

In addition to conflicts over landowner status and the delay of royalty payments, the 2017 national elections were plagued by violence, fraud, and coerced and bribed voting, with stuffed and stolen ballot boxes. Across the nation, including in Hela Province, more than two hundred people were killed during the election period, and many more were injured and maimed (*Guardian* 2018). Lingering animosities about contested and potentially fraudulent outcomes resulted in more violent conflicts.

Then, in February 2018, a magnitude 7.5 earthquake struck, and Hela Province was severely affected, with people, houses, fields, and sources of water covered over by landslides. In the aftermath,

> At least 18,000 people were displaced and living in informal camps or other evacuation facilities, often without adequate water and sanitation. Damaged airfields, bridges and roads, coupled with security threats related to inter-communal violence, complicated the response in some affected areas. A third of all health facilities in Hela and Southern Highlands Provinces closed in the immediate aftermath of the earthquake. (WHO 2018)

Friends of mine who were affected by these events said that armed gangs took advantage of the crisis to invade homes, hold up vehicles, rape women, and extort money for aid or transport. Warfare took place in and around Tari town itself, far worse than in the past because of the massive influx of high-powered weapons into the area. "Heavily armed clansmen interviewed during an outbreak of warfare in 2016 spoke of their several day journey from Komo to the West Papuan border, carrying 20kg rice bags that they had filled with marijuana grown for the exchange of weapons with Indonesia's armed forces," Jubilee Australia reported (Main and Fletcher 2018: 28). Threatened by gangs or enemy clans, and without a secure source of food, many women I knew fled the area, some to relatives who lived in remote areas not affected by fighting or the earthquake, and some as far away as urban settlements in Mendi or Mt. Hagen. There they often went into debt renting houses and agricultural land.

How these crises affected the HIV-positive women I interviewed, I do not know. Courageous hospital staff and nuns continued to provide care during Tari's earlier tumultuous period in the early 2000s, so I think it is quite likely that they did so again during this time. Whether patients have been able to make their way safely to places where they could receive their supplies of ARVs is another question. Having seen how flexible health workers were willing to be about "the rules" of ARVs, I have some confidence that they did their best to adapt to the situation and perhaps provided patients with more than the typical three-month supply for those who might face difficulties returning to the hospital or clinic.

GENDER AND AIDS IN TARI

In this book I have undertaken an expansive analysis of the "feminization of AIDS," showing how gender, as a relation of power, shapes all dimensions of HIV experience. Much like women around the world, women in Tari face specific vulnerabilities to infection. And while public health researchers often focus on female subjects' own risk behaviors, in many instances it would be more appropriate to examine how historical circumstances and structural relations of inequality put women in the path of others' risk behaviors. Where the state abandons responsibility, women find themselves vulnerable to crime, including sexual violence. When customary landowners, de facto defined as male, can display and consolidate their wealth and power by becoming patrons to men below them in the resource-extraction hierarchy, women may be "conned" into serving as tribute wives, making them vulnerable to a landowner husband's other sexual relationships.

Women's greater vulnerability to HIV, and their lesser ability to remove themselves from unsafe relationships and environments, is well documented. Less examined is how target audiences are interpellated as gendered subjects in AIDS interventions intended to enhance participants' consciousness about gender stereotypes and gender-based violence. These interventions may be done with the best of intentions, but they often treat gender as a culturally informed role rather than as a power relation thickly and inextricably enmeshed with other relations of power, especially in postcolonial contexts. In particular, the assumption that women are victims lacking agency may not reflect—indeed, may significantly distort –participants' more complex and nuanced understandings of gendered and other unequal social relations, including those in which men are disempowered, exploited, or silenced. The flattening of such complexities can alienate both participants and educators, who may consequently engage in translational agency, or even translational activism, thereby transforming or censoring problematic content. In the particular workshop I analyzed, the situation was further complicated by the way in which Huli women—but not Huli men—were cast as unhygienic subjects and sources of revulsion to health workers.

Finally, gendered relations of power also shape the experience of being HIV-positive. In this case, both material and discursive elements put women living with HIV in a tenuous position. That Huli women generally cannot act as custodians of clan land or owners of their own houses means that they are dependent on either a husband or natal kin to provide them with both shelter and land for cultivation. This material dependency for the most basic of needs has myriad consequences. For one thing, a few women ostracized by family were or had been homeless, a truly unheard-of situation in the past. And some who were living with the families of their adult siblings felt that they needed to prove both that they had labor value for the household and that they did not pose a health or social threat. Otherwise, they feared eviction. Those who lived alone felt that they were disproportionately vulnerable to theft, in part because they did not have men to protect them, but in part because thieves knew that HIV-positive women living alone were less likely to bring such disputes to village court. Finally, women's inability to claim clan land and houses as their own made it impossible for unrelated HIV-positive women to live together, and more generally meant that living with HIV was often a solitary experience for them, rather than something shared. These material precarities— which drove a couple of the women I interviewed to sell sex or cultivate other kinds of transactional sexual partnerships—were exacerbated by discourses that figure women as morally unreliable, inherently more duplicitous than men, and in need of externally imposed limits and rules. Thus, even women who were materially secure and loved by their families engaged in the gendered ethical work of allaying others' ungrounded fears and suspicions, treading a fine line between trying to live "like normal" and dispelling concerns that they might try to "pass" as "normal."

It should be noted that one might equally take up the issue of the "masculinization" of AIDS—that is, the ways in which gender as a relation of power has implications for men's experiences of HIV. For example, precisely because Huli men are the advantaged and dominant gender—and maleness is discursively constructed as self-disciplined, beautiful, purposeful, and pure (Wardlow 2006a)—there are strong expectations that men will "fence in" the household and not make it vulnerable to a fatal and stigmatized illness. When the male participants in the AIDS education workshop talked about the importance of being able to walk around "hands free," they made it clear that in public fora, men are always performing masculinity for other men, are acutely sensitive to how they might be perceived, and fear the consequences of not living up to other men's expectations of masculinity. Infecting one's wife with HIV, and one's children through maternal transmission, is a clear violation of the expectation that men will nurture and protect their households, and thus a powerful source of shame. Moreover, during the pre-antiretroviral era, when people sometimes asserted that God wanted to punish the HIV-positive person and "erase his lineage into the future," it was men suffering from AIDS that people had in mind, not women. And, as the custodians of clan land who should be able to pass their land on to their sons, it was men living with HIV who were most afraid that conniving kin would take advantage of their frail and stigmatized state to appropriate their territory and evict their children. Thus, it is perhaps not surprising that the few men I interviewed expressed a great deal more shame, guilt, and fear about being HIV-positive than the women I interviewed. It would seem that being the dominant gender can carry with it its own burdens, vulnerabilities, and terrors.

A FINAL WORD: THINKING ABOUT HIV
AND ARVS IN CONTEXT

There were a number of times during my interviews when I was struck by the fact that being HIV-positive was not the worst or most preoccupying of women's problems. As one means of assessing the stigma or opprobrium they faced, I asked women if they had anyone who would help them when the time came to build a new house, an expensive and laborious undertaking. Not worrying about this situation usually meant that a woman was well supported and anticipated being so in the future, while being very worried about this indicated isolation and abandonment. During one interview, a woman expressed concern about this, and when I followed up and asked whether she had brothers in the vicinity who might assist her, she replied that she'd had one brother, but he had been killed by her husband. She and her daughters had been living with her husband in Port Moresby, but returned home to the Tari area for what was supposed to be a short visit. While there, her oldest daughter, nine or ten at the time, was sexually assaulted, and her husband blamed her brother. The story, including the identity of the assailant, was a bit muddled, and I felt compelled to ask her whether it was her brother himself who had assaulted her daughter, or whether her husband blamed her brother because he had failed to protect her daughter when he was entrusted with her care. She at first indicated the former, then said she was unsure, and then didn't want to talk about it anymore.

In addition, it appeared that her brother had cashed in their plane tickets back to Port Moresby, and kept the money for himself, and so what was meant to be a short visit had turned into a very long stay. When her husband learned about his daughter's sexual assault, he came to Tari, tracked down her brother, and smashed his head in. As she put it, "He told me, 'Your brother obviously has no brains, so I removed them for him.'" As a consequence, her husband now refused to come back to Tari for fear that her kin would murder him in retaliation. And she had no intention of moving back to Port Moresby to be with him, because he had infected her with HIV, killed her brother, and remained angry with her because of her brother's actions. All this was in answer to why she worried that she had no one to help her build a new house. The challenges and preoccupations faced by other women I interviewed were not as dramatic as this woman's, but it was not unusual for their narratives to reveal relational and other issues that were of much greater concern to them than living with HIV.

HIV/AIDS policy makers often seem to assume that HIV is, or should be, at the forefront of the minds of people living with it, and that failure to demonstrate this might indicate that they are insufficiently attuned to "the rules" of being an AIDS patient. An alternative approach might view ARVs as enabling patients to feel well enough to deal with more pressing problems, just like any other medication. The view that people should prioritize their HIV vulnerability or their HIV patient-hood can be viewed as a form of AIDS exceptionalism detrimental to people whose lives are complicated by crime, patchy public services, unreliable economic opportunities, migration, election violence, fractious and violent kin relations, and so on. This book has sought to map the context that makes women in Tari vulnerable to HIV/AIDS in complexly gendered ways, but living with HIV is clearly only one of the challenges they face—and hardly the most fraught.

NOTES

INTRODUCTION

1. All names in this book are pseudonyms. In some instances other details, such as a person's place of residence, have also been changed in order to ensure confidentiality.

2. In 2013, the medical eligibility criteria for starting antiretroviral treatment in Papua New Guinea were a CD4 count of less than 350 or a combination of clinical symptoms associated with AIDS, such as wasting, chronic diarrhea, or atypical TB. In 2015, the treatment initiation guidelines were revised to a CD4 count of less than 500.

3. The tremendous happiness expressed by people over jobs should not be taken to mean that the LNG project was wholeheartedly embraced or viewed as entirely beneficial. Indeed, the project was considered so contentious that the final agreements for it were signed on an island about as far as you can get from Tari without being in another country, presumably to avoid Huli protestors' derailing the event.

4. Tari Hospital was still in a dismal state, so the narrow focus of the MSF project was also a source of confusion.

5. Two Papua New Guinean male university student interns were with me during this interview, and they later commented that whenever they came home from Port Moresby, for fear of its allure emanating from them attracting too many young women, their parents would not allow them to leave the house for a few days.

6. The research proposals were reviewed and approved by a number of different research ethics committees: the NIH (for the 2004 research), University of Toronto's Research Ethics Board, the Papua New Guinea National AIDS Council, and the Papua New Guinea Medical Research Advisory Committee.

7. This book draws primarily on the interviews with women. For work based primarily on the interviews with men, see Wardlow 2007, 2008, and 2014; Hirsch et al. 2010.

1. "RURAL DEVELOPMENT ENCLAVES"

1. This does not mean that Pamela was nine years old when she got married. Many children in the Tari area do not enroll in grade 1 until they are at least nine, and, in more rural areas, they may be as old as ten or eleven. Pamela was therefore likely around fifteen when she was married.

2. PJV became 95 percent owned and fully operated by Barrick Gold in 2006, when Barrick bought Placer Dome Inc. Currently, Barrick and Zijin Mining Group each own 47.5 percent of the operation, with the remaining 5 percent held by Mineral Resources Enga.

3. PMV stands for "public motor vehicle," and includes many types of vehicle, from buses to open flatbed trucks.

4. Kelly et al. (2011) found that landowners are the most common clients of sex workers in Port Moresby. The HIV prevalence among the groups interviewed was 19 percent among female sex workers, 8.8 percent among male sex workers, and 23.7 percent among transgender sex workers. Regular condom use was low. This particular study was done when business development grants and other payments were being distributed to PNG LNG Huli landowners, many of whom had migrated en masse to Port Moresby in anticipation of receiving these payments. So it is likely that many of the landowners discussed in Kelly et al. 2011 were Huli men.

5. Moreover, according to Human Rights Watch, the leadership of the Porgera Landowners Association, an organization formed to advocate for landowners' interests, "are thought by some to be lining their pockets with royalty payments that might otherwise flow to ordinary landowners. The PLOA is a well-resourced institution: in 2009, it received K3.6 million ($1.4 million) in royalty payments, a figure comparable in scale to the K4.5 million ($1.7 million) in royalties paid out in direct distributions to all of the SML's landowners that year. But there is no transparency as to how the organization spends its money. None of the landowners interviewed by Human Rights Watch—including several people on PLOA's board—had ever seen a detailed accounting of how the organization uses its financial resources" (Human Rights Watch 2011: 35).

6. In Papua New Guinea, fried "lamb flaps"—fatty, inexpensive, low-quality rib meat—are often sold as roadside fast food (see Gewertz and Errington 2010).

7. Newly diagnosed patients are still encouraged to "eat lots of fruit," so it is not surprising that when Kelapi heard this phrase, she immediately knew she was HIV-positive. The hospital worker in this story was probably afraid to reveal Kelapi's HIV status to her, because, assigned to a different department, he had no training in HIV counselling and could have been fired and taken to village court if Kelapi had responded to her HIV-positive status by killing herself.

8. Prevention of mother-to-child transmission (PMTCT) programs, drugs, and counseling were not available at that time, and even in 2013, when I completed this research, most of the women I interviewed did not know about these.

2. STATE ABANDONMENT, SEXUAL VIOLENCE, AND TRANSACTIONAL SEX

1. Médecins sans frontières perpetually worried that its project in Tari was treating only a small percentage of the victims of sexual violence in the area, and MSF staff asked me for my opinion as to why this was the case. I was surprised myself to discover that two years

after its establishment, many women's group leaders knew nothing about the MSF project at Tari Hospital. I repeatedly recommended that MSF reach out to the many highly organized church-affiliated women's groups in the area as the best way to ensure that women knew about the services it provided, but as employees of an NGO primarily involved in clinical care, MSF staff only seemed to feel comfortable doing outreach at health centers.

2. Sarah said that she had recently found purpose in comforting women who worried they might be HIV-positive and accompanying them when they went to be tested. She brightened up considerably when she talked about this. Nevertheless, I was concerned that she might try to kill herself, either out of despair about her future or in order to put in motion a compensation case against her mother, since it is common to demand compensation for suicide if it can be argued that the accused was a *tene*—that is, played some part in driving the person to it. I spoke with the clinic staff about monitoring her and gave her information about MSF's counselling services.

3. Papua New Guinea's tax credit scheme allows mining companies to use up to .75 percent of what they would owe in taxes for infrastructure projects.

4. The Melanesian Peace Foundation was the one exception, and their employees bravely spent weeks in the area trying to train people in negotiation skills that might prevent or end tribal fighting.

5. This gang had held up stores, kidnapped a political candidate, abducted young women from roadside markets, and invaded Tari High School, breaking into the girls' dormitory and kidnapping some of the female students.

6. Reporting increased somewhat after 2009, when MSF began offering counselling to survivors of sexual violence.

7. Huli women often wear two or more skirts, and refer to the underskirts as petticoats, a practice and terminology that must have been introduced by missionaries at some point.

8. By the time I returned in 2010, MSF had taken charge of all sexual violence cases, and the care it provided was entirely therapeutic in nature. Although it did occasionally make medical reports available if a woman herself requested it, it strongly resisted being "enrolled" (Callon 1986) into a network attempting to establish a "truth" about a young woman's sexual history.

3. LOVE, POLYGYNY, AND HIV

1. "You-statements" are often accusatory in nature and can escalate conflict—e.g., "You never listen to me!" In contrast, "I-statements" are aimed at sharing feelings—e.g., "When I feel that you aren't listening to me, I feel hurt."

2. See www.psi.org/publication/hiv-prevention-and-control-in-rural-development -enclaves-project-tokaut-na-tokstret-marital-relationship-training. Also see www.youtube .com/watch?v = 5OmIVzo5uEk which shows interviews with couples who have participated.

3. Neither the 2004 nor the later interviews were random samples, and I am thus not claiming that these proportions are representative. That said, epidemiological research elsewhere in the highlands of Papua New Guinea does indicate very high prevalence of sexually transmitted infections (Passey et al. 1998, Tiwara et al. 1996).

4. Evidence from sub-Saharan Africa (Reniers and Watkins 2010) suggests that polygyny may be a "benign" form of sexual concurrency, providing some protection from HIV, which underlines the importance of understanding polygyny in its lived social context.

4. TEACHING GENDER TO PREVENT AIDS

1. My calculus was correct. One night, a vehicle carrying food and supplies for Tari High School arrived very late, and it was decided that the safest place to store everything was in the police station just around the corner from where I was staying. Alerted to the delivery, a gang broke in, took the food, and stole police guns. Hearing the shooting, I blocked the doors to my guesthouse from the inside with whatever I could find (mostly a collection of derelict foot peddle sewing machines left over from some aborted women's development project). The gang sent a messenger to inform me that they had considered breaking in and stealing my belongings, but knew that I was carrying out AIDS education and providing free condoms and so decided not to. There were other factors that were probably more of a deterrent to them, such as not wanting to make an enemy of the woman who ran my guesthouse. Nevertheless, I was reassured to know that my efforts to provide a service had been noticed and counted in my favor.

2. PEPFAR's "90, 90, 90" refers to three specific goals: that by 2020, 90 percent of people living with HIV will know their status, 90 percent of those diagnosed HIV-positive will be receiving antiretroviral therapy, and 90 percent of those on antiretroviral therapy will have achieved viral suppression.

6. "LIKE NORMAL": THE ETHICS OF LIVING WITH HIV

1. Short sections of this chapter, particularly the discussions of hygienic morality and absolute candor, were previously published in the *Journal of the Royal Anthropological Institute* (Wardlow 2017), where I emphasize what I called HIV-positive women's (extra) ordinary ethics. This chapter, in contrast, emphasizes what Lisa Tessman (2005) calls the "burdened virtues" cultivated by women, and their attempts to live "like normal" but not be perceived as trying to "pass as normal."

2. What are called elementary schools in Tari are pre-schools intended to prepare children for primary school (grades 1–6) by teaching them to read and write in Huli. The theory is that it will be easier for children to become literate in English later if they have already studied their natal language. Many children enroll in grade 1 without having first attended an elementary school, and elementary school teachers are not required to have a formal teaching degree.

3. It is worth asking whether Huli have always felt this way, or whether rules and taboos acquired more force under colonial government. Many Huli assert, for example, that the Huli word *mana* should not be translated as "custom," as it is in many Huli-English dictionaries, but as "law." Australian colonial officers made a point of emphasizing the importance of "law and order"—and were well able to enforce these principles through fines, jail time, and forced labor. It's possible, I think, that in order to assert the equal value of Huli ethics, people might have emphasized their legalistic and disciplinary aspects. Alternatively, the sociopolitical changes wrought by the colonial period—and particularly, diminishing gerontocratic authority and the increasing autonomy of women and youth—might also have motivated senior men to emphasize the rule-oriented and disciplinary nature of Huli culture.

Abrams, Philip. 1988. "Notes on the Difficulty of Studying the State." *Journal of Historical Sociology* 1, no. 1: 58–89.

Aggleton, Peter, Stephen Bell, and Angela Kelly-Hanku. 2014. "'Mobile Men with Money': HIV Prevention and the Erasure of Difference." *Global Public Health* 9, no. 3: 257–70.

Ahmed, Sara. 2004. "Collective Feelings: Or, the Impressions Left by Others." *Theory, Culture & Society* 21, no. 2: 25–42.

———. 2010. *The Promise of Happiness.* Durham, NC: Duke University Press.

———. [2004] 2015. *The Cultural Politics of Emotion.* 2nd ed. New York: Routledge.

Allen, Bryant. 1995. "At Your Own Risk: Studying Huli Residency." In *Papuan Borderlands: Huli, Duna and Ipili Perspectives on the Papua New Guinea Highlands,* edited by Aletta Biersack, 141–72. Ann Arbor: University of Michigan Press.

Alpers, Philip. 2004. "Gun Violence, Crime and Politics in the Southern Highlands: Community Interviews and a Guide to Military-style Arms in Papua New Guinea." www.gunpolicy.org/fr/documents/5217-gun-violence-crime-and-politics-in-the-southern-highlands/file.

Amadiume, Ifi. 1987. *Male Daughters, Female Husbands: Gender and Sex in an African Society.* London: Zed Books.

Amstel, Hans van, and Sjaak van der Geest. 2004. "Doctors and Retribution: The Hospitalisation of Compensation Claims in the Highlands of Papua New Guinea." *Social Science & Medicine* 59, no. 10: 2087–94.

Andersen, Barbara. 2013. "Tricks, Lies, and Mobile Phones: 'Phone Friend' Stories in Papua New Guinea." *Culture, Theory and Critique* 54, no. 3: 318–34.

———. 2017. "Careful Words: Nursing, Language, and Emotion in Papua New Guinea." *Medical Anthropology: Cross Cultural Studies in Health and Illness* 36, no. 8: 758–71.

Appadurai, Arjun. 1988. "Putting Hierarchy in Its Place." *Cultural Anthropology* 3, no. 1: 36–49.

Aretxaga, Begoña. 2003. "Maddening States." *Annual Review of Anthropology* 32: 393–410.

Asian Development Bank [cited as ADB]. 2006a. "Grant Agreement for HIV/AIDS Prevention and Control in Rural Development Enclaves Project between the Independent State of Papua New Guinea and ADB." www.adb.org/projects/documents/grant-agreement -hiv-aids-prevention-and-control-rural-development-enclaves-project.

———. 2006b. "Proposed Asian Development Fund Grant Papua New Guinea: HIV/AIDS Prevention and Control in Rural Development Enclaves Project." www.adb.org/projects /documents/hiv-aids-prevention-and-control-rural-development-enclaves-project-rrp.

Ballard, Chris. 1994. "The Centre Cannot Hold: Trade Networks and Sacred Geography in the Papua New Guinea Highlands." *Archaeology in Oceania* 29, no. 3: 130–48.

Bargetz, Brigitte. 2015. "The Distribution of Emotions: Affective Politics of Emancipation." *Hypatia* 30, no. 3: 580–96.

Barker, Joshua, Eric Harms, and Johan Lindquist, eds. 2013. "Introduction." In *Figures of Southeast Asian Modernity*. Honolulu: University of Hawai'i Press.

Barss, Peter Geoffrey. 1991. "Health Impact of Injuries in the Highlands of Papua New Guinea: A Verbal Autopsy Study." PhD diss., Johns Hopkins University, School of Public Health.

Basu, Sanjay, David Stuckler, Gregg Gonsalves, and Mark Lurie. 2009. "The Production of Consumption: Addressing the Impact of Mineral Mining on Tuberculosis in Southern Africa." *Globalization and Health* 5, no. 11: 1–8.

Beckman, Nadine, and Janet Bujra. 2010. "The 'Politics of the Queue': The Politicization of People Living with HIV/AIDS in Tanzania." *Development and Change* 41, no. 6: 1041–64.

Benton, Adia, Thurka Sangaramoorthy, and Ippolytos Kalofonos. 2017. "Temporality and Positive Living in the Age of HIV/AIDS: A Multisited Ethnography." *Current Anthropology* 58, no. 4: 454–64.

Berlant, Lauren. 1998. "Intimacy: A Special Issue." *Critical Inquiry* 24, no. 2: 281–88.

———. 2011. *Cruel Optimism*. Durham, NC: Duke University Press.

Beyers, Christiaan. 2018. "Moral Subjectivity and Affective Deficit in the Transitional State: On Claiming Land in South Africa." In *Affective States: Entanglements, Suspensions, Suspicions*, edited by Mateusz Laszczkowski and Madeleine Reeves, 66–82. New York: Berghahn.

Biersack, Aletta. 1995. "Heterosexual Meanings: Society, Economy, and Gender among Ipilis." In *Papuan Borderlands: Huli, Duna, and Ipili Perspectives on the Papua New Guinea Highlands*, edited by A. Biersack, 231–63. Ann Arbor: University of Michigan Press.

———. 1999. "The Mt. Kare Python and His Gold: Totemism and Ecology in the Papua New Guinea Highlands." *American Anthropologist* 101, no. 1: 68–87.

———. 2001. "Dynamics of Porgera Gold Mining: Culture, Capital, and the State." In *Mining in Papua New Guinea: Analysis and Policy Implications*, edited by B. Imbun and P. McGavin, 25–44. Port Moresby: University of Papua New Guinea Press.

———. 2016. "Introduction: Emergent Masculinities in the Pacific." *Asia Pacific Journal of Anthropology* 17, nos. 3–4: 197–212.

Biersack, Aletta, Margaret Jolly, and Martha Macintyre, eds. 2016. *Gender Violence and Human Rights: Seeking Justice in Fiji, Papua New Guinea, and Vanuatu*. Canberra: Australian National University Press.

Bond, Virginia. 2010. "'It Is Not an Easy Decision on HIV, Especially in Zambia': Opting for Silence, Limited Disclosure and Implicit Understanding to Retain a Wider Identity." *AIDS Care* 22, no. S1: 6–13.

Bonnell, S. 1999. "Social Change in the Porgera Valley." In *Mining in Papua New Guinea: Analysis and Policy Implications*, edited by B. Imbun and P. McGavin, 19–87. Port Moresby: University of Papua New Guinea Press.

Borrey, Anou. 2000. "Sexual Violence in Perspective: The Case of Papua New Guinea." In *Reflections on Violence in Melanesia*, edited by Sinclair Dinnen and Allison Ley, 105–18. Canberra: Hawkins Press and Asia Pacific Press.

Braidotti, Rosi. 2002. *Metamorphoses: Towards a Materialist Theory of Becoming.* Cambridge: Polity Press.

Briggs, Charles. 2005. "Communicability, Racial Discourse, and Disease." *Annual Review of Anthropology* 34: 269–91.

Briggs, Charles, with Clara Mantini-Briggs. 2004. *Stories in the Time of Cholera: Racial Profiling during a Medical Nightmare.* Berkeley: University of California Press.

Buchanan, Holly, Frances Akuani, Francis Kupe, Angelyn Amos, Kayleen Sapak, Francis Be, Thomas Kawage, Rei Frank, and Murray Couch. 2011. *Behavioural Surveillance Research in Rural Development Enclaves in Papua New Guinea: A Study with the Oil Search Limited Workforce.* Papua New Guinea National Research Institute Special Publication Number 61. Boroko, Papua New Guinea: National Research Institute.

Burchardt, Marian. 2014. "The Logic of Therapeutic Habitus: Culture, Religion and Biomedical AIDS Treatments in South Africa." In *Religion and AIDS Treatment in Africa: Saving Souls, Prolonging Lives,* edited by Rijk van Dijk, Hansjörg Digler, Marian Burchardt, and Thera Rasing, 49–72. Burlington, VT: Ashgate.

Burnet, Jennie E. 2012. "Situating Sexual Violence in Rwanda (1990–2001): Sexual Agency, Sexual Consent, and the Political Economy of War." *African Studies Review* 55, no. 2: 97–118.

Callon, Michel. 1986. "Some Elements of a Sociology of Translation: Domestication of the Scallops and the Fishermen of St. Brieuc Bay." In *Power, Action and Belief: A New Sociology of Knowledge?* edited by J. Law, 196–223. London: Routledge.

Campbell, Catherine. 1997. "Migrancy, Masculine Identities and AIDS: The Psychosocial Context of HIV Transmission on the South African Gold Mines." *Social Science and Medicine* 45, no. 2: 273–81.

———. 2000. "Selling Sex in the Time of AIDS: the Psycho-social Context of Condom Use by Sex Workers on a Southern African Mine." *Social Science and Medicine* 50, no. 4: 479–94.

———. 2003. *Letting Them Die: Why HIV/AIDS Prevention Programs Fail.* Bloomington: Indiana University Press.

Card, Claudia. 1996. *The Unnatural Lottery: Character and Moral Luck.* Philadelphia: Temple University Press.

Castro, Arachu, and Paul Farmer. 2005. "Understanding and Addressing AIDS-Related Stigma: From Anthropological Theory to Clinical Practice in Haiti." *American Journal of Public Health* 95, no. 1: 53–59.

Clark, Jeffrey. 1993. "Gold, Sex, and Pollution: Male Illness and Myth at Mt. Kare, Papua New Guinea." *American Ethnologist* 20, no. 4: 742–57.

Colvin, Christopher, Steven Robins, and Joan Leavens. 2010. "Grounding 'Responsibilisation Talk': Masculinities, Citizenship and HIV in Cape Town, South Africa." *Journal of Development Studies* 46, no. 7: 1179–95.

Connell, John. 2005. *Papua New Guinea: The Struggle for Development.* New York: Routledge.

Corporate Social Responsibility Newswire. 2007. "Barrick Marks World AIDS Day with New Clinics in PNG and Tanzania." *CSR News,* November 30, 2007, www.csrwire.com /press_releases/16007-Barrick-Marks-World-AIDS-Day-with-New-Clinics-in-PNG -and-Tanzania.

Crush, Jonathan, Brian Williams, Eleanor Gouws, and Mark Lurie. 2005. "Migration and HIV/AIDS in South Africa." *Development Southern Africa* 22, no. 3: 293–318.

Crush, Jonathan, Ines Raimundo, Hamilton Simelane, Boaventura Cau, and David Dorey. 2010. *Migration-Induced HIV and AIDS in Rural Mozambique and Swaziland.* Waterloo, ON: Southern African Migration Policy Series No. 53. Cape Town: Southern African Research Centre.

Cullen, Trevor. 2006. "HIV/AIDS in Papua New Guinea: A Reality Check." *Pacific Journalism Review* 12, no. 1: 155–66.

Cvetkovich, Ann. 2012. *Depression: A Public Feeling.* Durham, NC: Duke University Press.

Das, Veena. 1996. "Sexual Violence, Discursive Formations and the State." *Economic and Political Weekly* 31, nos. 35–37: 2411–23.

———. 2015. "What Does Ordinary Ethics Look Like?" In M. Lambek, V. Das, D. Fassin, and W. Keane, *Four Lectures on Ethics: Anthropological Perspectives,* 53–125. Chicago: HAU Books.

Das, Veena, and Deborah Poole. 2004. "The State and Its Margins: Comparative Ethnographies." In *Anthropology in the Margins of the State,* edited by Veena Das and Deborah Poole, 3–34. Santa Fe, NM: School of American Research Press.

Desmond, Nicola, Caroline Allen, Simon Clift, Butolwa Justine, Joseph Msugu, Mary Plummer, Deborah Watson-Jones, and David Ross. 2005. "A Typology of Groups at Risk of HIV/STI in a Gold Mining Town in North-Western Tanzania." *Social Science and Medicine* 60: 1739–49.

Dilger, Hansjörg. 2001. "'Living PositHIVely in Tanzania': The Global Dynamics of AIDS and the Meaning of Religion for International and Local AIDS Work." *Afrika Spectrum* 36, no. 1: 73–90.

Dilger, Hansjörg, Marian Burchardt, and Rijk van Dijk. 2014. "Introduction: Religion and AIDS Treatment in Africa: The Redemptive Moment." In *Religion and AIDS Treatment in Africa: Saving Souls, Prolonging Lives,* edited by Rijk van Dijk, Hansjörg Digler, Marian Burchardt, and Thera Rasing, 1–24. Burlington, VT: Ashgate.

Dinnen, Sinclair and Allison Ley, eds. 2000. *Reflections on Violence in Melanesia.* Canberra: Hawkins Press and Asia Pacific Press.

Donham, Donald L., with Santu Mofokeng. 2011. *Violence in a Time of Liberation: Murder and Ethnicity at a South African Gold Mine, 1994.* Durham, NC: Duke University Press.

Dorpar, Joseph, and Jim Macpherson. 2007. "The National Government and the Southern Highlands since the 2002 Elections." In *Conflict and Resource Development in the Southern Highlands of Papua New Guinea,* edited by N. Haley and R. J. May, 21–33. Canberra: ANU E Press.

Dundon, Alison. 2007. "Warrior Women, the Holy Spirit and HIV/AIDS in Rural Papua New Guinea." *Oceania* 77, no. 1: 29–42.

Enloe, Cynthia. 2000. *Maneuvers: The International Politics of Militarizing Women's Lives.* Berkeley: University of California Press.

Ernst, Thomas.1999. "Land, Stories, and Resources: Discourse and Entification in Onabasulu Modernity." *American Anthropologist* 101, no. 1: 88–97.

Esacove, Anne. 2016. *Modernizing Sexuality: U.S. HIV Prevention in Sub-Saharan Africa.* Oxford: Oxford University Press.

Eves, Richard. 2003. "AIDS and Apocalypticism: Interpretations of the Epidemic from Papua New Guinea." *Culture, Health & Sexuality* 5, no. 3: 249–64.

———. 2010. "Masculinities Matter." In *Civic Insecurity: Law, Order and HIV in Papua New Guinea,* edited by V. Luker and S. Dinnen, 47–79. Canberra: ANU E Press.

———. 2012. "Resisting Global AIDS Knowledges: Born-Again Christian Narratives of the Epidemic from Papua New Guinea." *Medical Anthropology* 31, no. 1: 61–76.

Fassin, Didier. 2015. Introduction: Toward a Critical Moral Anthropology. In *A Companion to Moral Anthropology,* edited by D. Fassin, 1–17. Malden, MA: Wiley Blackwell.

Ferguson, James. 2005. "Seeing Like an Oil Company: Space, Security, and Global Capital in Neoliberal Africa." *American Anthropologist* 107, no. 3: 377–82.

Filer, Colin. 1998. "The Melanesian Way of Menacing the Mining Industry." In *Modern Papua New Guinea,* edited by L. Zimmer-Tamakoshi, 147–78. Kirksville, MO: Thomas Jefferson University Press.

———. 2001. "Between a Rock and a Hard Place: Mining Projects, 'Indigenous Communities,' and Melanesian States." In *Mining in Papua New Guinea: Analysis and Policy Implications,* edited by B. Imbun and P. McGavin, 7–24. Port Moresby: University of Papua New Guinea Press.

Filer, Colin, and Benedict Imbun. 2004. *A Short History of Mineral Development Policies in Papua New Guinea.* Resource Management in Asia-Pacific Working Paper No. 55. Canberra: Research School of Pacific and Asian Studies, Australian National University.

Filer, Colin, and Martha Macintyre. 2006. "Grass Roots and Deep Holes: Community Responses to Mining in Melanesia." *The Contemporary Pacific* 18, no. 2: 215–31.

Filer, Colin, Siobhan McDonnell, and Matthew G. Allen. 2017. "Powers of Exclusion in Melanesia." In *Kastom, Property and Ideology: Land Transformations in Melanesia,* edited by S. McDonnell, M. G. Allen, and C. Filer, 1–55. Canberra: ANU Press. https://press.anu .edu.au/publications/series/state-society-and-governance-melanesia/kastom-property -and-ideology.

Fitzpatrick, P. 1980. "Really Rather Like Slavery: Law and Labor in the Colonial Economy in Papua New Guinea." *Contemporary Crises* 4, no. 1: 77–95.

Flora, Janne. 2012. "'I Don't Know Why He Did It. It Happened by Itself'": Causality and Suicide in Northwest Greenland." In *The Anthropology of Ignorance: An Ethnographic Approach,* edited by C. High, A. Kelly, and J. Mair, 137–62. New York: Palgrave.

Frankel, Stephen. 1980. "I Am Dying of Man." *Culture, Medicine, and Psychiatry* 4: 95–117.

———. 1986. *The Huli Response to Illness.* Cambridge: Cambridge University Press.

Gallagher, Kevin, and Lyuba Zarsky. 2007. *The Enclave Economy: Foreign Investment and Sustainable Development in Mexico's Silicon Valley.* Cambridge, MA: MIT Press.

Gebrekristos, Hirut, Stepehn Resch, Khangelani Zuma, and Mark Lurie. 2005. "Estimating the Impact of Establishing Family Housing on the Annual Risk of HIV Infection in South African Mining Communities." *Sexually Transmitted Diseases* 32, no. 6: 333–40.

Gershon, Ilana, and Dhooleka Sarhadi Raj. 2000. "Introduction: The Symbolic Capital of Ignorance." *Social Analysis: The International Journal of Social and Cultural Practice* 44, no. 2: 3–14.

Gewertz, Deborah, and Frederick Errington. 2010. *Cheap Meat: Flap Food Nations in the Pacific Islands.* Berkeley: University of California Press.

Giddens, Anthony. 1992. *The Transformation of Intimacy: Sexuality, Love, and Eroticism in Modern Societies.* Stanford, CA: Stanford University Press.

Gilberthorpe, Emma. 2007. "Fasu Solidarity: A Case Study of Kin Networks, Land Tenure, and Oil Extraction in Kutubu, Papua New Guinea." *American Anthropologist* 109, no. 1: 101–12.

Glasse, Robert M. 1968. *Huli of Papua: A Cognatic Descent System.* Paris: Mouton.

———. 1974. "Le Masque de la volupté: Symbolisme et antagonisme sexuels sur les hauts plateaux de Nouvelle-Guinée." *L'Homme* 14, no. 2: 79–86.

Goffman, Erving. 1963. *Stigma: Notes on the Management of Spoiled Identity.* New York: Simon & Schuster.

Goldman, Laurence. 1983. *Talk Never Dies: The Language of Huli Disputes.* London: Tavistock Publications.

Golub, Alex. 2006. "Who Is the 'Original Affluent Society'? Ipili 'Predatory Expansion' and the Porgera Gold Mine, Papua New Guinea." *The Contemporary Pacific* 18, no. 2: 265–92.

———. 2007a. "From Agency to Agents: Forging Landowner Identities in Porgera: Customary Land Tenure and Registration in Australia and Papua New Guinea." In *Customary Land Tenure and Registration in Australia and Papua New Guinea,* edited by J. Weiner and K. Glaskin, 73–96. Canberra: ANU E Press.

———. 2007b. "Ironies of Organization: Landowners, Land Registration, and Papua New Guinea's Mining and Petroleum Industry." *Human Organization* 66, no. 1: 38–48.

———. 2014. *Leviathans at the Gold Mine: Creating Indigenous and Corporate Actors in Papua New Guinea.* Durham, NC: Duke University Press.

Good, Kenneth. 1986. *Papua New Guinea: A False Economy.* London: Antislavery Society.

The Guardian. 2018. "Unprecedented Violence and Fraud 'Hijacked' 2017 PNG Election." October 30. www.theguardian.com/world/2018/oct/30/unprecedented-violence-and -hijacked-2017-png-election-report.

Haley, Nicole. 2007. "Cosmology, Morality and Resource Development: SHP Election Outcomes and Moves to Establish a Separate Hela Province." In *Conflict and Resource Development in the Southern Highlands of Papua New Guinea,* edited by N. Haley and R. J. May, 57–68. Canberra: ANU E Press.

Haley, Nicole, and Ronald J. May. 2007. "Introduction: Roots of Conflict in the Southern Highlands." In *Conflict and Resource Development in the Southern Highlands of Papua New Guinea,* edited by N. Haley and R. J. May, 1–19. Canberra: ANU E Press.

Haley, Nicole, and Robert Muggah. 2006. "Jumping the Gun? Reflections on Armed Violence in Papua New Guinea." *African Security Review* 15, no. 2: 38–55.

Halperin, Daniel, and Helen Epstein. 2004. "Concurrent Sexual Partnerships Help to Explain Africa's High HIV Prevalence: Implications for Prevention." *Lancet* 364, no. 9428 (July 3): 4–6.

Hammar, Lawrence. 2010. *Sin, Sex and Stigma: A Pacific Response to HIV and AIDS.* Wantage, England: Sean Kingston Publishing.

Hansen, Michael. 2014. "From Enclave to Linkage Economies?: A Review of the Literature on Linkages between Extractive Multinational Corporations and Local Industry in Africa." Copenhagen: Danish Institute for International Studies Working Paper. http://pure.diis.dk/ws/files/45256/wp2014_02_Michael_Hansen_for_web.pdf.

Hardon, Anita. 2012. "Biomedical Hype and Hopes: AIDS Medicine for Africa. In *Rethinking Biomedicine and Governance in Africa: Contributions from Anthropology,* edited by Paul Wenzel Geissler, Richard Rottenburg, and Julia Zenker, 77–96. Berlin: De Gruyter.

Hardon, Anita, and Deborah Posel. 2012. "Secrecy as Embodied Practice: Beyond the Confessional Imperative." *Culture, Health & Sexuality* 14, no. S1: 1–13.

Harman, Sophie. 2011. "The Dual Feminisation of HIV/AIDS." *Globalizations* 8, no. 2: 213–28.

Harris, Geoff T. 1972. "Labour Supply and Economic Development in the Southern Highlands." *Oceania* 43, no. 2: 123–39.

Hengehold, Laura. 2000. "Remapping the Event: Institutional Discourses and the Trauma of Rape." *Signs* 26, no. 1: 189–214.

High, Casey. 2012. "Between Knowing and Being: Ignorance in Anthropology and Amazonian Shamanism." In *The Anthropology of Ignorance: An Ethnographic Approach,* edited by C. High, A. Kelly, and J. Mair, 119–35. New York: Palgrave.

Hinton, Rachael, and Jaya Earnest. 2010. "'I Worry So Much I Think It Will Kill Me': Psychosocial Health and the Links to the Conditions of Women's Lives in Papua New Guinea." *Health Sociology Review* 19, no. 1: 5–19.

Hirsch, Jennifer, and Holly Wardlow, eds. 2006. *Modern Loves: The Anthropology of Romantic Courtship and Companionate Marriage.* Ann Arbor: University of Michigan Press.

Hirsch, Jennifer, Holly Wardlow, Daniel Smith, Shanti Parikh, Harriet Phinney, and Constance Nathanson. 2010. *The Secret: Love, Marriage, and HIV.* Nashville, TN: Vanderbilt University Press.

Howse, Genevieve. 2008. "Accessing Rights and Protections Under the HIV/AIDS Management and Prevention Act in Papua New Guinea: Making a Case for Granting a Limited Jurisdiction to the Village Courts.": *Journal of South Pacific Law* 12, no. 1: 1–16.

Human Rights Watch. 2011. "Gold's Costly Dividend: Human Rights Impacts of Papua New Guinea's Porgera Gold Mine." www.hrw.org/report/2011/02/01/golds-costly-dividend/human-rights-impacts-papua-new-guineas-porgera-gold-mine.

———. 2015. "Bashed Up: Family Violence in Papua New Guinea." www.hrw.org/report/2015/11/04/bashed/family-violence-papua-new-guinea.

Hunter, Mark. 2015. "The Political Economy of Concurrent Partners: Toward a History of Sex-Love-Gift Connections in the Time of AIDS." *Review of African Political Economy* 42, no. 145: 362–75.

Inbun, Benedict. 2006. "Local Laborers in Papua New Guinea Mining: Attracted or Compelled to Work?" *The Contemporary Pacific* 18, no. 2: 315–33.

Jacka, Jerry. 2001. "On the Outside Looking In: Attitudes and Responses of Non-Landowners Towards Mining at Porgera." In *Mining in Papua New Guinea: Analysis and Policy Implications,* edited by B. Imbun and P. McGavin, 45–62. Port Moresby: University of Papua New Guinea Press.

———. 2015. *Alchemy in the Rain Forest: Politics, Ecology, and Resilience in a New Guinea Mining Area.* Durham, NC: Duke University Press.

Jaggar, Alison. 1989. Love and Knowledge: Emotion in Feminist Epistemology. *Inquiry* 32: 151–176.

Johnson, Peter. 2010. *Lode Shedding: A Case Study of the Economic Benefits to the Landowners, the Provincial Government, and the State from the Porgera Gold Mine*. National Research Institute Discussion Paper 124.

Jolly, Margaret. 2000. "Epilogue: Further Reflections on Violence in Melanesia." In *Reflections on Violence in Melanesia*, edited by S. Dinnnen and A. Ley, 305–24. Sydney: Hawkins Press and Asia Pacific Press.

——. 2012. "Introduction–Engendering Violence in Papua New Guinea: Persons, Power and Perilous Transformations." In *Engendering Violence in Papua New Guinea*. edited by Margaret Jolly, Christine Stewart, and Carolyn Brewer, 1–46. Canberra: Australian National University Press.

——. 2016. "Men of War, Men of Peace: Changing Masculinities in Vanuatu." *Asia Pacific Journal of Anthropology* 17, nos. 3–4: 305–23.

Jolly, Margaret, Christine Stewart, and Carolyn Brewer, eds. 2012. *Engendering Violence in Papua New Guinea*. Canberra: Australian National University Press.

Jorgensen, Dan. 2001. "Who and What Is a Landowner? Mythology and Marking the Ground in a Papua New Guinea Mining Project." In *Emplaced Myth: Space, Narrative, and Knowledge in Aboriginal Australia and Papua New Guinea*, edited by A. Rumsey and J. Weiner, 101–24. Honolulu: University of Hawai'i Press.

Kaler, Amy, Nicole Angotti, and Astha Ramaiya. 2016. "'They Are Looking Just the Same': Antiretroviral Treatment as Social Danger in Rural Malawi." *Social Science & Medicine* 161 (October): 71–78

Kelly-Hanku, Angela, Martha Kupul, Wing Young Nicola Man, Somu Nosi, Namarola Lote, Patrick Rawstorne, Grace Halim, Claire Ryan and Heather Worth. 2011. "Askim na Save (Ask and Understand): People Who Sell and Exchange Sex in Port Moresby." Papua New Guinea Institute of Medical Research and the University of New South Wales. https://sphcm.med.unsw.edu.au/sites/default/files/sphcm/Centres_and_Units/Askim_na_Save.pdf.

Kelly-Hanku, Angela, Peter Aggleton, and Patti Shih. 2014. "'We Call It a Virus but I Want to Say It's the Devil Inside': Redemption, Moral Reform and Relationships with God among People Living with HIV in Papua New Guinea." *Social Science & Medicine* 119 (October): 106–13.

Kelly-Hanku, Angela, H. Aeno, L. Wilson, R. Eves, Agnes Mek, R. Nake Trumb, M. Whittaker, L. Fizgerald, J.M. Kaldor, and A. Vallely. 2016. "Transgressive Women Don't Deserve Protection: Young Men's Narratives of Sexual Violence against Women in Rural Papua New Guinea." *Culture, Health & Sexuality* 18, no. 11: 1207–20.

Koivunen, Anu. 2010. An Affective Turn? Reimagining the Subject of Feminist Theory. In *Working with Affects in Feminist Readings: Disturbing Differences*, edited by M. Liljeström and S. Paasonen, 8–29. New York: Routledge.

Krupa, Christopher, and David Nugent. 2015. "Off-Centred States: Rethinking State Theory through an Andean Lens." In *State Theory and Andean Politics: New Approaches to the Study of Rule*, edited by C. Krupa and D. Nugent, 1–31. Philadelphia: University of Pennsylvania Press.

Laidlaw, James. 2002. "For an Anthropology of Ethics and Freedom." *Journal of the Royal Anthropological Institute* 8, no. 2 (June): 311–32.

Lambek, Michael. 2010a. "Introduction." In *Ordinary Ethics: Anthropology, Language, and Action,* edited by M. Lambek, 1–36. New York: Fordham University Press.

———. 2010b. "Toward an Ethics of the Act." In *Ordinary Ethics: Anthropology, Language, and Action,* edited by M. Lambek, 39–63. New York: Fordham University Press.

Laszczkowski, Mateusz, and Madeleine Reeves. 2018. "Introduction: Affect and the Anthropology of the State." In *Affective States: Entanglements, Suspensions, Suspicions,* edited by Mateusz Laszczkowski and Madeleine Reeves, 1–14. New York: Berghahn.

Lavu, Kai. 2007. "Porgera Joint Venture's Presence in the Southern Highlands Province." In *Conflict and Resource Development in the Southern Highlands of Papua New Guinea,* edited by N. Haley and Ron J. May, 129–34. Canberra: ANU E Press.

Lederman, Rena. 1986. *What Gifts Engender: Social Relations and Politics in Mendi, Highland Papua New Guinea.* Cambridge: Cambridge University Press.

Lehmann, Deborah. 2002. "Demography and Causes of Death among the Huli in the Tari Basin." *Papua New Guinea Medical Journal* 45, nos. 1–2 (March): 51–62.

Lehmann, Deborah, John Vail, Joe Crocker, Helen Pickering, Michael Alpers, and the Tari Demographic Surveillance Team. 1997. "Demographic Surveillance in Tari, Southern Highlands Province, Papua New Guinea: Methodology and Trends in Fertility and Mortality between 1979–1993." Goroka: Papua New Guinea Institute of Medical Research.

Lepani, Katherine. 2008. "Mobility, Violence and the Gendering of HIV in Papua New Guinea." *Australian Journal of Anthropology* 19, no. 2: 150–64.

Levy, Jennifer, and Katerini Storeng. 2007. "Living Positively: Narrative Strategies of Women Living with HIV in Cape Town, South Africa." *Anthropology and Medicine* 14, no. 1: 55–68.

Lewis, Ione, Bessie Maruia, and Sharon Walker. 2008. "Violence against Women in Papua New Guinea." *Journal of Family Studies* 14, nos. 1–2: 183–97.

Li, Tania Murray. 2007. *The Will to Improve: Governmentality, Development, and the Practice of Politics.* Durham, NC: Duke University Press.

Liamputtong, Pranee, Niphattra Haritavorn, and Niyada Kiatying-Angsulee. 2009. "HIV and AIDS, Stigma and AIDS Support Groups: Perspectives from Women Living with HIV and AIDS in Central Thailand." *Social Science & Medicine* 69, no. 6: 862–68.

Lorde, Audre. 1984. *Sister Outsider: Essays and Speeches.* Trumansburg, NY: Crossing Press.

Lutz, Catherine. 1995. "The Gender of Theory." In *Women Writing Culture,* edited by Ruth Behar and Deborah Gordon, 249–66. Berkeley: University of California Press.

Lyttleton Chris. 2004. "Fleeing the Fire: Transformation and Gendered Belonging in Thai HIV/AIDS Support Groups." *Medical Anthropology* 23, no. 1: 1–40.

Macintyre, Martha. 2008. "Police and Thieves, Gunmen and Drunks: Problems with Men and Problems with Society in Papua New Guinea." *Australian Journal of Anthropology* 19, no. 2: 179–93.

Mah, Timothy, and Daniel Halperin. 2010. "Concurrent Sexual Partnerships and the HIV Epidemics in Africa: Evidence to Move Forward." *AIDS and Behavior* 14, no. 1: 11–16.

Mahmood, Saba. 1995. *Politics of Piety: The Islamic Revival and the Feminist Subject.* Princeton, NJ: Princeton University Press.

Main, Michael, and Luke Fletcher. 2018. "On Shaky Ground: PNG LNG and the Consequences of Development Failure." Jubilee Australia report. Sydney: Jubilee Australia Research Centre.

Mair, Jonathan, Ann Kelly, and Casey High. 2012. "Introduction: Making Ignorance and Ethnographic Object. In *The Anthropology of Ignorance: An Ethnographic Approach*, edited by C. High, A. Kelly, and J. Mair, 1–32. New York: Palgrave.

Malinowski, Bronislaw. 1922. *Argonauts of the Western Pacific*. London: Routledge.

Mama, Amina. 1997. "Sheroes and Villains: Conceptualizing Colonial and Contemporary Violence against Women in Africa." In *Feminist Genealogies, Colonial Legacies, Democratic Futures*, edited by Jacqui Alexander and Chandra T. Mohanty, 46–62. New York: Routledge.

Mannell, Jenevieve. 2010. "Gender Mainstreaming Practice: Considerations for HIV/AIDS Community Organisations." *AIDS Care* 22 (supplement 2): 1613–19.

Marks, Shula. 2006. "The Silent Scourge? Silicosis, Respiratory Disease and Gold-Mining in South Africa." *Journal of Ethnic and Migration Studies* 32, no. 4: 569–89.

Mattes, Dominik. 2011 "'We Are Just Supposed to Be Quiet': The Production of Adherence to Antiretroviral Treatment in Urban Tanzania." *Medical Anthropology* 30, no. 2: 158–82.

———. 2012. "'I Am Also a Human Being!': Antiretroviral Treatment in Local Moral Worlds." *Anthropology and Medicine* 19, no. 1: 75–84.

———. 2014. "Caught in Transition: the Struggle to Live a 'Normal' Life with HIV in Tanzania." *Medical Anthropology* 33, no. 4 (January): 270–87.

Mattingly, Cheryl. 2014. *Moral Laboratories: Family Peril and the Struggle for a Good Life*. Berkeley: University of California Press.

McGavin, Paul A., LukeT. Jones, and Benedict Y. Imbun. 2001. "In Country Fly-In/Fly-Out and National HR Development: Evidence from Papua New Guinea." In *Mining in Papua New Guinea: Analysis and Policy Implications*, edited by Benedict Y. Imbun and Paul A. McGavin. Port Moresby: University of Papua New Guinea Press.

McIlraith, James, Sarah Robinson, Lily Lesley Pyrambone, Luke Petai, Darchiney Sinebare, and Sylvia Maipa. 2012. *The Community Good: Examining the Influence of the PNG LNG Project in the Hela Region of Papua New Guinea. Report sponsored by ChildFund Australia, the New Zealand National Centre for Peace and Conflict Studies, the PNG Church Partnership Programme, Oxfam Highlands Programme, Jubilee Australia, and the Melanesian Institute.* Otago, NZ: University of Otago.

McKenzie, Fiona. 2010. "Fly-In Fly-Out: The Challenges of Transient Populations in Rural Landscapes." In *Demographic Change in Australia's Rural Landscapes: Implications for Society and the Environment*, edited by G. Luck, R. Black, and D. Race, 353–74. Landscape Series, vol. 12. Dordrecht: Springer.

Mcleod, Abby, and Marth Macintyre. 2010. "The Royal Constabulary." In *Civic Insecurity: Law, Order and HIV in Papua New Guinea*, edited by V. Luker and S. Dinnen. Canberra: ANU E Press.

Médecins sans frontières [cited as MSF]. 2011. *Hidden and Neglected: The Medical and Emotional Needs of Survivors of Family and Sexual Violence in Papua New Guinea.* www.doctorswithoutborders.org/sites/usa/files/06–15-Papua-New-Guinea-Sexual-Domestic-Violence%20report.pdf.

Meger, Sara. 2010. "Rape of the Congo: Understanding Sexual Violence in the Conflict in the Democratic Republic of Congo." *Journal of Contemporary African Studies* 28, no. 2: 119–35.

Meinert, Lotte, Hanne Mogensen, and Jenipher Twebaze. 2009. "Tests for Life Chances: CD4 Miracles and Obstacles in Uganda." *Anthropology and Medicine* 16, no. 2: 195–209.

Merry, Sally Engle. 2006. *Human Rights and Gender Violence: Translating International Law into Local Justice*. Chicago: University of Chicago Press.

Mfecane, Sakhumzi. 2011. "Negotiating Therapeutic Citizenship and Notions of Masculinity in a South African Village." *African Journal of AIDS Research* 10, no. 2: 129–38.

Mgone, Charles, Megan Passey, Joseph Anang, Wilfred Peter, Tony Lupiwa, Dorothy Russell, Diro Babona, and Michael Alpers. 2002. "Human Immunodeficiency Virus and Other Sexually Transmitted Infections among Female Sex Workers in Two Major Cities in Papua New Guinea." *Sexually Transmitted Diseases* 29, no. 5: 265–70.

Moffett, Helen. 2006. "'These Women, They Force Us to Rape Them': Rape as Narrative of Social Control in Post-Apartheid South Africa." *Journal of Southern African Studies* 32, no. 1: 129–44.

Mohanty, Chandra. 1984. "Under Western Eyes: Feminist Scholarship and Colonial Discourses." *boundary 2* 12, no. 3: 333–58.

Mukherjee, Aprajita, and Madhumita Das. 2011. "Mainstreaming Gender in HIV Programs: Issues, Challenges and Way Forward." *Eastern Journal of Medicine* 16: 153–59.

Mulla, Sameena. 2014. *The Violence of Care: Rape Victims, Forensic Nurses, and Sexual Assault Intervention*. New York: New York University Press.

Nagel, Thomas. 1993. "Moral Luck." In *Moral Luck,* edited by Daniel Statman, 57–71. Albany: State University of New York Press.

Navaro-Yashin, Yael. 2002. *Faces of the State: Secularism and Public Life in Turkey*. Princeton, NJ: Princeton University Press.

Ngai, Sianne. 2005. *Ugly Feelings*. Cambridge. MA: Harvard University Press.

Nguyen, Vinh-Kim. 2008. "Antiretroviral Globalism, Biopolitics, and Therapeutic Citizenship." In *Global Assemblages: Technology, Politics, and Ethics as Anthropological Problems,* edited by Aiwa Ong and Stephen J. Collier, 124–44. Oxford: Blackwell.

———. 2013. "Counselling against HIV in Africa: A Genealogy of Confessional Technologies." *Culture, Health & Sexuality* 15 (July): S440–52.

Nnaemeka, Obioma. 2004. "Nego-Feminism: Theorizing, Practicing, and Pruning Africa's Way." *Signs* 29, no. 2: 357–85.

Oyewumi, Oyeronke. 1997. *The Invention of Women: Making an African Sense of Western Gender Discourses*. Minneapolis: University of Minnesota Press.

Packard, Randall. 1989. *White Plague, Black Labour: Tuberculosis and the Political Economy of Health and Disease in South Africa*. Berkeley: University of California Press.

Papua New Guinea National AIDS Council [cited as PNG NAC]. 2006. *Papua New Guinea National Strategic Plan on HIV / 2006–2010*. Port Moresby: PNG NAC.

———. 2007. *Introduction to HIV and AIDS: Participant's Manual*. Port Moresby: National AIDS Council Secretariat.

———. 2010. *Papua New Guinea National HIV and AIDS Strategy, 2011–2015*. Port Moresby: PNG NAC.

———. 2014. Papua New Guinea Interim Global AIDS Response Progress & Universal Access Report.

Parker, Richard, and Peter Aggleton. 2003. "HIV and AIDS-related Stigma and Discrimination: A Conceptual Framework and Implications for Action." *Social Science & Medicine* 57, no. 1 (July): 13–24.

Parla, Ayse. 2001. "The 'Honor' of the State: Virginity Examinations in Turkey." *Feminist Studies:* 27, no. 1: 65–88.

Passey, Megan, Charles Mgone, N. Suve, S. Tiwara, Tony Lupiwa, A. Clegg, and Michael Alpers. 1998. "Community Based Study of Sexually Transmitted Diseases in Rural Women in the Highlands of Papua New Guinea: Prevalence and Risk Factors." *Sexually Transmitted Disease* 74, no. 2 (April): 120–27.

Paudel, Vikas, and Kedar Baral. 2015. "Women Living with HIV/AIDS (WLHA), Battling Stigma, Discrimination and Denial and the Role of Support Groups as a Coping Strategy: A Review of Literature." *Reproductive Health* 12, no. 53. https://preview-reproductive-health-journal.biomedcentral.com/articles/10.1186/s12978-015-0032-9.

Porgera Environmental Advisory Committee [cited as PEAK]. 2011. "Scoping Project: Social Impact of the Mining Project on Women in the Porgera Area." Penny Johnson, Consultant.

Pedwell, Carolyn, and Anne Whitehead. 2012. "Affecting Feminism: Questions of Feeling in Feminist Theory." *Feminist Theory* 13, no. 2: 115–29.

Pigg, Stacy. 2001. "Languages of Sex and AIDS in Nepal: Notes on the Social Production of Commensurability." *Cultural Anthropology* 16, no. 4: 481–541.

———. 2005. "Globalizing the Facts of Life." In *Sex in Development: Science, Sexuality, and Morality in Global Perspective,* edited by V. Adams and S. Pigg, 39–65. Durham, NC: Duke University Press.

Pinker, Annabel, and Penny Harvey. 2015. "Negotiating Uncertainty: Neo-liberal Statecraft in Contemporary Peru." In *Affective States: Entanglements, Suspensions, Suspicions,* edited by Mateusz Laszczkowski and Madeleine Reeves, 15–31. New York: Berghahn.

Population Services International. 2013. Gender-Based Violence and Marital Relations Training Facilitators' Guide (draft).

Pratt, Geraldine, and Victoria Rosner. 2012. "Introduction." In *The Global and the Intimate: Feminism in Our Time,* edited by G. Pratt and V. Rosner, 1–27. New York: Columbia University Press.

Prince, Ruth. 2012. "The Politics and Anti-Politics of HIV Interventions in Kenya." In *Rethinking Biomedicine and Governance in Africa: Contributions from Anthropology,* edited by Paul Wenzel Geissler, Richard Rottenburg, and Julia Zenker, 97–116. Berlin: De Gruyter.

Rajak, Dinah. 2011. *In Good Company: An Anatomy of Corporate Social Responsibility.* Stanford, CA: Stanford University Press.

Rand, Erin. 2015. "Bad Feelings in Public: Rhetoric, Affect, and Emotion." *Rhetoric and Public Affairs* 18, no. 1: 161–75.

Rasmussen, Louise Mubanda. 2014. "Negotiating Holistic Care with the 'Rules' of ARV Treatment in A Catholic Community-Based Organization in Kampala." In *Religion and AIDS Treatment in Africa: Saving Souls, Prolonging Lives,* edited by Rijk van Dijk, Hansjörg Dilger, Marian Burchardt, and Thera Rasing, 247–70. Burlington, VT: Ashgate.

Redman-MacLaren, Michelle, Jane Mills, Rachael Tommbe, David MacLaren, Richard Speare, and William McBride. 2013. "Women and HIV in a Moderate Prevalence Setting: An Integrative Review." *BMC Public Health* 13: 552–65.

Reniers, George, and Susan Watkins. 2010. "Polygyny and the Spread of HIV in Sub Saharan Africa: A Case of Benign Concurrency." *AIDS* 24, no. 2: 299–307.

Rhine, Kathryn A. 2009. "Support Groups, Marriage, and the Management of Ambiguity among HIV-Positive Women in Northern Nigeria." *Anthropology Quarterly* 82, no. 2 (Spring): 369–400.

Rix, Anne. 2018. ExxonMobil's Public and Government Affairs public response to concerns about the ExxonMobil liquid natural gas project in Papua New Guinea. www.business-humanrights.org/en/papua-new-guinea-lack-of-project-benefits-by-exxonmobil-and-oil-search-escalate-violence-within-project-communities.

Robbins, Joel. 2004. "The Globalization of Pentecostal and Charismatic Christianity." *Annual Review of Anthropology* 33: 117–43.

Robins, Steven. 2006. "From 'Rights' to 'Ritual': AIDS Activism in South Africa." *American Anthropologist* 108, no. 2: 312–23.

Roscoe, Paul. 2014. "The End of War in Papua New Guinea: 'Crime' and 'Tribal Warfare' in Post-Colonial States." *Anthropologica* 56, no. 2: 327–39.

Schieffelin, Edward. 1983. "Anger and Shame in the Tropical Forest: On Affect as a Cultural System in Papua New Guinea." *Ethos* 11, no. 3: 181–191.

Scott, James C. 1998. Seeing Like a State: How Certain Schemes to Improve the Human Condition Have Failed. New Haven, CT: Yale University Press.

Sedgewick, Eve. 2003. *Touching Feeling: Affect, Pedagogy, Performativity.* Durham, NC: Duke University Press.

Seeley, Janet, and Kate Butcher. 2006. "'Mainstreaming' HIV in Papua New Guinea: Putting Gender Equity First." *Gender & Development* 14, no. 1: 105–14.

Seifert, Ruth. 1994. "War and Rape: A Preliminary Analysis." In *Mass Rape: The War against Women in Bosnia-Herzegovina,* edited by A. Stiglmayer, 54–72. Lincoln: University of Nebraska Press.

Shand, Tim, Haley Thomson-de Boor, Wessel van den Berg, Laura Peacock, and Dean Pascoe. 2014. "The HIV Blind Spot: Men and HIV Testing, Treatment and Care in sub-Saharan Africa." *IDS Bulletin* 1, 53–60.

Shih, Patti, Heather Worth, Joanee Travaglia, and Angela Kelly-Hanku. 2017. "'Good Culture, Bad Culture': Polygyny, Cultural Change and Structural Drivers of HIV in Papua New Guinea." *Culture, Health & Sexuality* 19, no. 9: 1024–1037.

Spelman, Elizabeth. 1989. "Anger and Insubordination." In *Women, Knowledge, and Reality,* edited by A. Garry and M. Pearsall, 263–73. Boston: Unwin Hyman.

Spronk, Rachel. 2009. "Media and the Therapeutic Ethos of Romantic Love in Middle-Class Nairobi." In *Love in Africa,* edited by J. Cole and L. Thomas, 181–203. Chicago. University of Chicago Press.

Stead, Victoria. 2017. "Landownership as Exclusion." In *Kastom, Property and Ideology: Land Transformations in Melanesia,* edited by S. McDonnell, Matthew G. Allen, and C. Filer, 357–81. Canberra: ANU Press. https://press.anu.edu.au/publications/series/state-society-and-governance-melanesia/kastom-property-and-ideology.

Steady, Filomina Chioma. 1987. "African Feminism: A Worldwide Perspective." In *Women in Africa and the African Diaspora,* edited by Rosalyn Terborg-Penn, Sharon Harley, and Andrea Benton Rushing, 3–24. Washington, DC: Howard University Press.

Stewart, Christine. 2012. "'Crime to be a Woman?': Engendering Violence against Female Sex Workers in Port Moresby, Papua New Guinea." In *Engendering Violence in Papua New Guinea,* edited by M. Jolly, C. Stewart, and C. Brewer, 213–38. Canberra: Australian National University Press.

Stewart, R. G. 1992. *Coffee: The Political Economy of an Export Industry in Papua New Guinea.* Boulder, CO: Westview Press.

Storey, Keith. 2001. "Fly-in/Fly-out and Fly-over: Mining and Regional Development in Western Australia." *Australian Geographer* 32, no. 2: 133–48.

Strathern, Andrew. 1971. *Rope of Moka: Big-Men and Ceremonial Exchange in Mount Hagen New Guinea.* Cambridge: Cambridge University Press.

———. 1975. "Why Is Shame on the Skin?" *Ethnology* 14, no. 4: 347–56.

———. 1982. "The Division of Labor and Processes of Social Change in Mount Hagen." *American Ethnologist* 9, no. 2: 307–19.

Strathern, Marilyn. 1979. "The Self in Self-Decoration." *Oceania* 49, no. 4: 241–57.

———. 1988. *The Gender of the Gift: Problems with Women and Problems with Society in Melanesia.* Berkeley: University of California Press.

Street, Alice. 2012. "Seen by the State: Bureaucracy, Visibility and Governmentality in a Papua New Guinean Hospital." *Australian Journal of Anthropology* 23, no. 1 (April): 1–21.

———. 2014. *Biomedicine in an Unstable Place: Infrastructure and Personhood in a Papua New Guinea Hospital.* Durham, NC: Duke University Press.

Tavory, Iddo, and Ann Swidler. 2009. "Condom Semiotics: Meaning and Condom Use in Rural Malawi." *American Sociological Review* 74, no. 2: 171–89.

Tessman, Lisa. 2000. "Moral Luck in the Politics of Personal Transformation." *Social Theory and Practice* 26, no. 3: 375–95.

———. 2001. "Critical Virtue Ethics: Understanding Oppression as Morally Damaging." In *Feminists Doing Ethics,* edited by P. DesAutels and Joanne Waugh, 79–100. Boulder, CO: Rowman & Littlefield.

———. 2005. *Burdened Virtues: Virtue Ethics for Liberatory Struggles.* Oxford: Oxford University Press.

Tiwara, S. Megan Passey, A. Clegg, Charles Mgone, S. Lupiwa, N. Suve, and Tony Lupiwa. 1996. "High Prevalence of Trichomonal Vaginitis and Chlamydial Cervicitis among a Rural Population in the Highlands of Papua New Guinea." *Papua New Guinea Medical Journal* 39: 234–38.

Thornberry, Elizabeth. 2015. "Virginity Testing History, and the Nostalgia for Custom in Contemporary South Africa." *African Studies Review* 58, no. 3: 129–48.

Ticktin, Miriam. 2011. "The Gendered Human of Humanitarianism: Medicalising and Politicising Sexual Violence." *Gender and History* 23, no. 2: 250–65.

Toft, Susan, ed. 1985. *Domestic Violence in Papua New Guinea.* Monograph No. 3, Law Reform Commission of Papua New Guinea.

Turshen, Meredeth. 2001. "The Political Economy of Rape: An Analysis of Systematic Rape and Sexual Abuse of Women During Armed Conflict in Africa." In *Victors, Perpetrators or Actors: Gender, Armed Conflict and Political Violence,* edited by C. Mose and F. Clarke, 55–68. London: Zed Books, 2001.

Tymoczko, Maria. 2010. "Translation, Resistance, Activism: An Overview." In *Translation, Resistance, Activism,* edited by Maria Tymoczko, 1–22. Amherst: University of Massachusetts Press.

UNAIDS. 2010. "Papua New Guinea Releases New HIV Prevalence Estimates." www.unaids.org/en/resources/presscentre/featurestories/2010/august/20100826fspng.

United Nations. General Assembly. Special Session on HIV/AIDS [cited as UNGASS]. 2008. *UNGASS 2008 Country Progress Report: Papua New Guinea: Reporting Period, January 2006–December 2007.* Port Moresby: PNG National AIDS Council Secretariat.

United States. President's Emergency Plan for AIDS Relief [cited as PEPFAR]. 2016. *Papua New Guinea Country Operation Plan (COP) 2016 Strategic Direction Summary.* www .state.gov/wp-content/uploads/2019/08/Papua-New-Guinea-9.pdf.

Vail, John. 1995. "All that Glitters: the Mt. Kare Goldrush and its Aftermath. In *Papuan Borderlands: Huli, Duna, and Ipili Perspectives on the Papua New Guinea Highlands,* edited by A. Biersack, 343–74. Ann Arbor: University of Michigan Press.

——. 2007. "Community-Based Development in Tari—Present and Prospects." In *Conflict and Resource Development in the Southern Highlands of Papua New Guinea,* edited by N. Haley and R. J. May, 101–21. Canberra: ANU E Press.

Varga, Christine. 1997. "The Condom Conundrum: Barriers to Condom Use among Commercial Sex Workers in Durban, South Africa." *African Journal of Reproductive Health / La Revue Africaine de la Santé Reproductive* 1, no. 1: 74–88.

Venuti, Lawrence. 2008. *The Translator's Invisibility: A History of Translation.* 2nd ed. New York: Routledge.

Vogler, Candace. 1998. "Sex and Talk." *Critical Inquiry* 24, no. 2: 328–65.

Ward, R. Gerard. 1990. Contract Labor Recruitment from the Highlands of Papua New Guinea 1950–1974. *International Migration Review* 24, no. 2: 273–96.

Wardlow, Holly. 1996. "Bobby Teardrops: A Turkish Video in Papua New Guinea. Reflections on Cultural Studies, Feminism, and the Anthropology of Mass Media." *Visual Anthropology Review* 12, no. 1: 30–46.

——. 2001. "The Mt. Kare Python: Huli Myths and Gendered Fantasies of Agency." In *Mining and Indigenous Life Worlds in Australia and Papua New* Guinea, edited by Alan Rumsey and James Weiner, 31–67. Adelaide, Australia: Crawford House Press.

——. 2002. "Headless Ghosts and Roving Women: Specters of Modernity in Papua New Guinea." *American Ethnologist* 29, no. 1: 5–32.

——. 2004. "Anger, Economy, and Female Agency: Problematizing 'Prostitution' and 'Sex Work' in Papua New Guinea." *Signs: Journal of Women in Culture and Society* 29, no. 4: 1017–40.

——. 2006a. *Wayward Women: Sexuality and Agency in a New Guinea Society.* Berkeley: University of California Press.

——. 2006b. "All's Fair when Love Is War: Romantic Passion and Companionate Marriage among the Huli of Papua New Guinea." In *Modern Loves: The Anthropology of Romantic Courtship and Companionate Marriage,* edited by J. Hirsch and H. Wardlow, 51–77. Ann Arbor: University of Michigan Press.

——. 2007. "Men's Extramarital Sexuality in Rural Papua New Guinea." *American Journal of Public Health* 97, no. 6: 1006–14.

——. 2008. "'She Liked It Best when She Was on Top': Intimacies and Estrangements in Huli Men's Marital and Extramarital Relationships." In *Intimacies: Love and Sex across Cultures,* edited by William Jankowiak, 194–223. New York: Columbia University Press.

——. 2009. "Labour Migration and HIV Risk in Papua New Guinea." In *Mobility, Sexuality and AIDS,* edited by Mary Haour-Knipe, Peter Aggleton, and Felicity Thomas, 176–86. New York: Routledge.

——. 2012. "The Task of the HIV Translator: Transforming Global AIDS Knowledge in an Awareness Workshop." *Medical Anthropology* 31, no. 5: 404–19.

——. 2014. "Paradoxical Intimacies: The Christian Creation of the Huli Domestic Sphere." In *Divine Domesticities: Christian Paradoxes in Asia and the Pacific,* edited by

Hyaeweol Choi and Margaret Jolly, 325–44. Canberra: Australian National University Press.

———. 2017. "The (Extra)ordinary Ethics of Being HIV-positive in Rural Papua New Guinea." *Journal of the Royal Anthropological Institute* 23, no. 1: 103–19.

———. 2018. "HIV, Phone Friends, and Affective Technology in Papua New Guinea." In *The Moral Economy of Mobile Phones in the Pacific,* edited by Robert Foster and Heather Horst, 39–52. Canberra: Australian National University Press.

Wardlow, Holly, and Jennifer Hirsch. 2006. "Introduction." In *Modern Loves: The Anthropology of Romantic Courtship and Companionate Marriage,* edited by J. Hirsch and H. Wardlow, 1–31. Ann Arbor: University of Michigan Press.

Welker, Marina. 2016. "No Ethnographic Playground: Mining Projects and Anthropological Politics, a Review Essay." *Comparative Studies in Society and History* 58, no. 2: 577–86.

West, Paige. 2012. *From Modern Production to Imagined Primitive: The Social World of Coffee from Papua New Guinea.* Durham, NC: Duke University Press.

White, Joanna, and John Morton. 2005. "Mitigating Impacts of HIV/AIDS on Rural Livelihoods: NGO Experiences in sub-Saharan Africa." *Development in Practice* 15, no. 2: 186–99.

Williams, Bernard. 1981. *Moral Luck.* New York: Cambridge University Press.

Wilson, Ara. 2004. *The Intimate Economies of Bangkok: Tomboys, Tycoons, and Avon Ladies in the Global City.* Berkeley: University of California Press.

———. 2012. "Intimacy: A Useful Category of Transnational Analysis." In *The Global and the Intimate: Feminism in Our Time,* edited by G. Pratt and V. Rosner, 31–56. New York: Columbia University Press.

World Health Organisation [cited as WHO]. 2004. *HIV/AIDS in Asia and the Pacific Region 2003.* Manila: World Health Organization, Western Pacific–South-East Asia.

———. 2018. "Papua New Guinea Earthquake." www.who.int/westernpacific/emergencies/papua-new-guinea-earthquake.

Zigon, Jared. 2009. "Morality and Personal Experience: The Moral Conceptions of a Muscovite Man." *Ethos* 37, no. 1 (March): 78–101.

Zimmer-Tamakoshi, Laura. 2012. "Troubled Masculinities and Gender Violence in Melanesia." In *Engendering Violence in Papua New Guinea,* edited by C. Jolly, C. Stewart, and C. Brewer, 73–106. Canberra: Australian National University Press.

Founded in 1893,
UNIVERSITY OF CALIFORNIA PRESS
publishes bold, progressive books and journals
on topics in the arts, humanities, social sciences,
and natural sciences—with a focus on social
justice issues—that inspire thought and action
among readers worldwide.

The UC PRESS FOUNDATION
raises funds to uphold the press's vital role
as an independent, nonprofit publisher, and
receives philanthropic support from a wide
range of individuals and institutions—and from
committed readers like you. To learn more, visit
ucpress.edu/supportus.